The Healthy

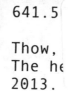

Morag Thow, PhD, BSc, Dip PE, MCSP, MBE

Keri Graham, MCSP, MSc, BSc (Hons)

Choi Lee, BSc (Hons), RD

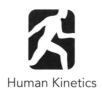

Human Kinetics

Library of Congress Cataloging-in-Publication Data

Thow, Morag K.
  The healthy heart book / Morag Thow, PhD, BSc, Dip PE, MCSP, MBE, Keri Graham MCSP, MSc, BSc (Hons), Choi Lee, BSc (Hons) RD.
    pages cm
  Includes index.
  1. Heart--Diseases--Diet therapy--Recipes. 2. Low-cholesterol diet--Recipes. 3. Coronary heart disease--Prevention. I. Graham, Keri, 1974- II. Lee, Choi, 1975- III. Title.
  RC684.D5T46 2013
  641.5'6311--dc23
                              2012050491

ISBN-10: 1-4504-3278-6 (print)
ISBN-13: 978-1-4504-3278-8 (print)

Developmental Editor: Anne Hall; **Assistant Editor:** Tyler M. Wolpert; **Copyeditor:** Joanna Hatzopoulos Portman; **Indexer:** Laurel Plotzke; **Permissions Manager:** Martha Gullo; **Graphic Designer:** Nancy Rasmus; **Graphic Artist:** Kim McFarland; **Cover Designer:** Keith Blomberg; **Photograph (cover):** Photodisc/Getty Image; **Photographs (interior):** © Human Kinetics, unless otherwise noted; **Photo Asset Manager:** Laura Fitch; **Visual Production Assistant:** Joyce Brumfield; **Photo Production Manager:** Jason Allen; **Art Manager:** Kelly Hendren; **Associate Art Manager:** Alan L. Wilborn; **Illustrations:** © Human Kinetics, unless otherwise noted; **Printer:** Versa Press

Human Kinetics books are available at special discounts for bulk purchase. Special editions or book excerpts can also be created to specification. For details, contact the Special Sales Manager at Human Kinetics.

Printed in the United States of America   10   9   8   7   6   5   4   3   2   1

The paper in this book is certified under a sustainable forestry program.

Human Kinetics
Website: www.HumanKinetics.com

United States: Human Kinetics
P.O. Box 5076
Champaign, IL 61825-5076
800-747-4457
e-mail: humank@hkusa.com

Canada: Human Kinetics
475 Devonshire Road Unit 100
Windsor, ON N8Y 2L5
800-465-7301 (in Canada only)
e-mail: info@hkcanada.com

Europe: Human Kinetics
107 Bradford Road
Stanningley
Leeds LS28 6AT, United Kingdom
+44 (0) 113 255 5665
e-mail: hk@hkeurope.com

Australia: Human Kinetics
57A Price Avenue
Lower Mitcham, South Australia 5062
08 8372 0999
e-mail: info@hkaustralia.com

New Zealand: Human Kinetics
P.O. Box 80
Torrens Park, South Australia 5062
0800 222 062
e-mail: info@hknewzealand.com

E5744

The Healthy Heart Book

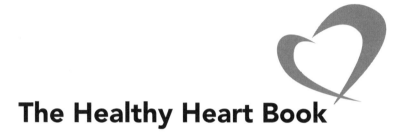

Morag Thow, PhD, BSc, Dip PE, MCSP, MBE

Keri Graham, MCSP, MSc, BSc (Hons)

Choi Lee, BSc (Hons), RD

Contents

Foreword

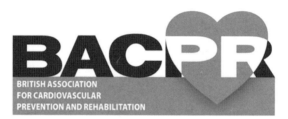

Promoting excellence in cardiovascular disease prevention and rehabilitation

So often, health and rehabilitation programmes provide people with heart disease with numerous leaflets and handouts that easily get misplaced and appear to have a short-life. Having a single, long lasting "proper" book that includes most of the written heart information resources under one cover literally gives it a long shelf-life, which can then be referred to as and when needed.

You may be someone who has experienced a heart problem, or you might have a family member or friend with heart disease. There are few books available for people like you that help you learn how to best cope with these conditions. Yet the number of books written for medical and health care professionals on heart health and rehabilitation is almost uncountable. The words and guidance in these many professional books are only of use if they can be transformed into helping you to understand and make changes for better health. Having a "how to" book for people like you, which reflects the work of heart health and rehabilitation practitioners, seems only logical.

The British Association for Cardiovascular Prevention and Rehabilitation (BACPR) is pleased to see that such a book, *The Healthy Heart Book*, is now available for people with heart disease and their families. This book reflects the core components set out by the BACPR for an effective heart health and rehabilitation programme. Literally, "at the heart" of these core components is helping people better understand your needs and make changes towards a healthier life. This means understanding and better managing lifestyle (activity, diet, smoking), mental and emotional well-being, medications, and so becoming your own health manager.

Success in anything, including being healthier and happier, is always best achieved when you have been able to take control and do it for yourself. This book can help you take the important guidance from the heart health team and transform it into your own heart health programme.

Preface

The Healthy Heart Book explains why and how to protect your heart with a healthy lifestyle. It also helps you to make sense of how and what you are feeling after a heart event such as heart attack, angina, stent insertion or heart surgery. After a heart event you may feel physically and emotionally overwhelmed; it can be frightening for you and those close to you. However, you are not alone. Each year, thousands of people are sharing the same experience. It is reassuring to know that, with the help of a healthy lifestyle, a large proportion of these people move on to live normal, healthy lives. In 2010 the British Heart Foundation (BHF) reported that over 56 thousand patients took part in health related cardiac rehabilitation in England, Northern Ireland and Wales. They reported the following year that there had been major improvements in survival rates following a heart event. If patients stick with a *healthy heart* lifestyle, they significantly increase their chance of longer, healthy lives. Many people take their health for granted, so when a heart event occurs it knocks their confidence. They think, *What? It can't be me!* This type of experience can change the way you think about your body. This book helps you understand that your thoughts and feelings are natural, teaches you to recognise when you need a bit more support, and ultimately gives you the tools to get control of your life.

In the pages of this book you will discover the following:

- What coronary heart disease is and how it is treated
- How you feel emotionally and physically after a heart event
- How a 'heart MOT' can help you assess your risk of coronary heart disease
- How to be active and exercise
- How to eat well for optimal heart health
- How to cope with stress and learn to relax
- How to access a wide range of sources of support
- How to continue to manage your healthy lifestyle in the long term

Each chapter provides examples of real-life experiences and easy, practical tips to help you on your way to a happy, healthy and confident future. Whether you or someone close to you has had heart ill-health or would like to find out more about a healthy lifestyle, this book is for you.

Introduction

You may already know of many things that you can do for your heart health. However, as is true for most people, what you *know* and what you *do* may not necessarily be connected. This book can help you make that connection.

If you have had a heart event, such as heart attack, angina, stent insertion or heart surgery, your physician has probably recommended that you begin a healthy heart programme, often referred to as cardiac rehabilitation. Ideally this programme includes doctors, nurses, physiotherapy and exercise specialists, dietitians and psychologists. This team helps you do the following:

- Understand your heart condition and how to best maintain the benefits of the medical treatments and therapies you have received
- Become more physically active in a safe, confident and enjoyable way
- Eat an enjoyable, healthy and balanced diet
- Stop smoking
- Manage feelings of stress, anxiety and depression related to your health and everyday life
- Understand the importance of your medication
- Continue to manage your healthy lifestyle in the long term

After a heart event, a big part of your recovery comes from you. However, you also benefit from the support of the medical profession and those closest to you. A healthy heart programme helps you gain confidence, motivation, fitness, knowledge and understanding. It is a valuable source of supervised exercise and education from supportive specialist professionals who help you take control of your life.

This book is a supplement to the support you receive from your local cardiac rehabilitation professionals. It helps you to understand what coronary heart disease is, the common feelings (emotional and physical) that people have after a diagnosis of heart disease, and what you can do to help yourself. It combines information about the most recent scientific evidence, expert opinion about heart health and, most important, the patient's and his or her loved ones' experiences. It is honest, useful and full of real-life stories.

When I was in hospital after having my heart attack I felt foolish and scared. I also thought, Why me? My head was a mess.

Danny, age 58

This book introduces all of the lifestyle changes you should consider making, if you haven't already, after a heart event. These changes include stopping smoking, living an active lifestyle and taking regular exercise, eating a healthy diet, keeping to a healthy weight and shape, making sensible choices about alcohol, and using effective coping strategies for negative feelings, stress, worry, anger and tension. The book offers practical ideas on how to protect your heart and how you and your loved ones can achieve improved heart health, improved general well-being, and a happy and confident future. For many people, having a heart event can literally change their lives. It encourages people to look at their lives and decide what is important and it motivates them to make positive changes in lifestyle. It can be a chance to have a more positive and fulfilling future.

My stent and the fright I had was the best thing that happened to me. I am now much fitter and I spend much more fun time with my grandchildren.

Hilda, age 62

This book reveals the honest journey of real-life cardiac patients. It gives you and your loved ones practical ways to take control and live a healthier life. It supports you during all the stages of your recovery. You can use it in your own time whenever you need to build and reinforce your healthy future.

For information that is beyond the scope of the book, we direct you to websites and other sources of support and information. References are carefully selected to help lead you to legitimate sources and dispel any common myths about heart health.

A Comprehensive Approach to Recovery

The British Association for Cardiovascular Prevention and Rehabilitation (BACPR) provides, develops and improves core standards to ensure the safe and effective delivery of cardiovascular prevention and rehabilitation practices and programmes throughout the UK. The following diagram demonstrates that the BACPR places equal emphasis on the delivery of care in the following areas: lifestyle risk factor management, psychosocial health, medical risk factor management and cardioprotective therapies.

This book covers all the core components necessary for a healthy heart and lifestyle. The BACPR diagram (figure 1) also indicates that health behaviour change and education are important to all the other components necessary for a healthy heart.

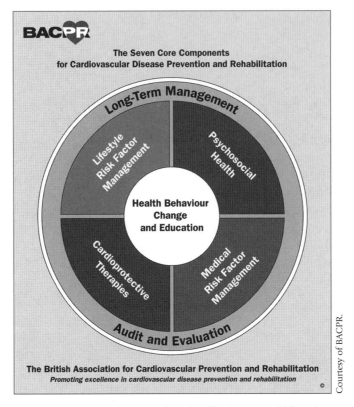

Figure 1 BACPR principles for a healthy heart and lifestyle.

Health behaviour change means how you go about changing unhealthy ways and habits. Each person is different, so when you decide to make changes in your own unique lifestyle, you need to understand why and how to make them for yourself. This book provides you with the education you need in order to make beneficial and life-long lifestyle decisions.

If you would like to know more information about the BACPR, see www.bacpr.com.

Coronary Heart Disease and How It Is Treated

Before we talk about your recovery from a heart event, let's have a quick look at a few questions you may be asking:

- What is coronary heart disease (CHD)?
- How does CHD affect the heart?
- How can CHD be treated?

This chapter answers these questions so that you can better understand what CHD is and how it is treated. It explains how the blood vessels that supply your heart muscle can become narrowed or blocked, how this change affects your heart, what symptoms it can cause and how it can be treated with medication and surgery.

Your heart is a fantastic organ (see figure 1.1). It is basically a muscular pump that can beat more than 100,000 times a day. Your heart pushes blood round your body to supply it with oxygen and nutrients.

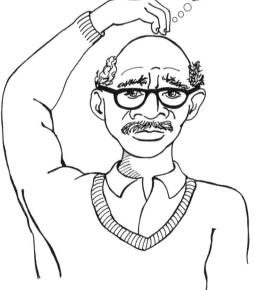

CHD, MI, angina, coronary arteries, angiogram, stent, bypass surgery— it's a foreign language!

It also receives a supply of vital, oxygen-rich blood. A large blood vessel, called the aorta, carries blood from the heart to the body. Close to where the aorta leaves the heart, small blood vessels, called coronary arteries, branch off and feed back into the heart muscle. Each time the heart beats, about 4 to 5 percent of the blood being pumped is pushed into the coronary arteries and supplies the heart itself; the rest goes round the body.

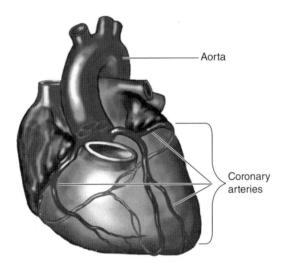

Figure 1.1   The coronary arterial system.

Defining Coronary Heart Disease (CHD)

Coronary heart disease (CHD) occurs when the inside of the wall of the coronary artery is damaged. Damaged sections in the inner wall of the artery start to become coated with fatty fibrous material that starts to clog up the artery. This material is called fatty plaque.

Fatty plaque takes up space inside the artery and therefore less space exists for blood to flow through the artery. Consequently, the blood flow to the part of the heart muscle being supplied by that artery is reduced. This reduction in oxygen-rich blood flow can cause symptoms called angina. The damage to the inside of the artery wall causes inflammation in the artery, potentially causing the fatty plaque to burst. When the fatty plaque bursts, a blood clot forms and it can block the blood flow completely. If the coronary artery is blocked completely, a heart attack can occur.

Picture This

Imagine that the hosepipe is your coronary artery, the water is blood and the grass is your heart. Pretend it's a good summer and there hasn't been any rain for a long time.

- You run a hosepipe into your garden to supply your grass with water.
- Grit starts to damage the inside of the hosepipe and it becomes rough in places. Dirt starts to gather at the rough area and the hosepipe is narrowed.
- Less water is flowing and the grass begins to suffer (angina).
- If the hosepipe blocks completely there will be no water supply and the grass will wither (heart attack).
- If the pipe is blocked for a very short period and the water starts flowing again quickly, the grass can recover (which is what happens if you get to hospital quickly).
- The longer the pipe is blocked, the more grass that is affected. If the pipe is blocked for a longer time, then some of the grass will die and never recover (damage to the heart muscle).

Angina

The narrowing effect of CHD reduces blood flow to the heart and can cause angina. Angina is the name given to the many symptoms that people feel when the heart isn't getting enough blood supply and therefore not enough oxygen is getting to the heart. Angina is the heart's way of telling you it needs more oxygen. Medical professionals often call angina *chest pain,* but many people do not feel pain. People feel angina in various ways and it can be severe or mild. All of this is confusing. Let's clear up the confusion by looking at many of the ways that you can feel angina.

How Can Angina Feel?

Discomfort in the centre of the chest

Heaviness or tightness in the chest

A dull ache in the chest

Heartburn or indigestion

Heaviness across the front of one or both shoulders

Pain or heaviness in one or both arms

Discomfort in the jaw

Heaviness in the throat

Discomfort between the shoulder blades

Undue or unexpected shortness of breath*

*If you have a lung condition and you are struggling to tell the difference between your lung symptoms and potential heart symptoms, discuss this with your doctor, practice nurse or cardiac rehabilitation professional.

Remember, there are lots of other things that can cause these symptoms, it might not be angina, but if you think it might be then use your GTN spray or tablets and discuss it with your doctor, practice nurse or cardiac rehabilitation team.

What to Do if You Think You Are Having Angina
If you have these symptoms and you think it could be angina, then take these steps:

1. Stop what you are doing.

2. Sit down, relax and take a few slow, deep breaths.

3. If you have a glyceryl trinitrate* (GTN) spray or tablet, use it under your tongue in the way your doctor, cardiac rehabilitation professional or pharmacist taught you. Guidelines would suggest that you take the spray and wait 5 minutes, then if your symptoms have not gone away take the spray again and wait 5 minutes. Then, if your symptoms have not gone away, call for an ambulance.

4a. If your symptoms have gone away within 15 minutes, it has not done any harm. However, you should discuss it with your doctor or cardiac rehabilitation professional. It may be possible to change the dosage or type of your medication to stop you from having angina.

4b. If your symptoms have not gone away within 15 minutes, phone for an ambulance *immediately* and stay resting until it arrives.

5. If you are not allergic to aspirin and someone is there to help you, chew an adult aspirin tablet (300 mg). Chewing, rather than swallowing the tablet whole, gets the medicine into your bloodstream faster. If you don't have an aspirin or you don't know if you are allergic to it, just stay sitting until the ambulance arrives.

*Glyceryl trinitrate (GTN) spray is a medicine that you spray under your tongue to relieve angina. Some people have GTN tablets instead. The tablets also go under your tongue and can be removed when your angina symptoms go away. If you have a GTN spray or tablet and you're not sure how much you should use, then you must speak with your doctor, practice nurse or cardiac rehab team immediately.

There are some common myths and misconceptions about angina (see table 1.1), so learning about these myths will help you understand angina further.

TABLE 1.1   **Common Myths and Facts About Angina**

Common myth or misconception	Fact
Angina is like a small heart attack.	Angina does not damage your heart if it subsides with rest or with use of glyceryl trinitrate (GTN) and lasts no more than 15 min.
If I use my GTN and the feeling I had wasn't angina, I'll do myself harm.	The effects of GTN last for only 30 min. It can give you a headache or make you feel a little lightheaded, but if used properly it cannot cause you any harm.
My symptoms are only a bit uncomfortable. It's not that bad, so I should wait until it gets bad.	People are used to putting up with a certain amount of pain (they wait until a headache is bad before they take pain killers). However, angina is different; if you feel it you must treat it immediately.
I can become dependent on GTN.	GTN is not addictive and you cannot become dependent on it.

Heart Attack

When a coronary artery is blocked completely and suddenly, causing the area of the heart muscle normally supplied by that artery to be starved of blood and oxygen, this area of heart muscle can be damaged. This event is called a heart attack, also known as a myocardial infarction (MI). A heart attack can feel just like angina: the symptoms can be quite mild or intense and severe. If you are having a heart attack, you might feel tightness, heaviness or pain in your chest, which may spread to your arms, neck, jaw, back or stomach. Some people who are having a heart attack feel short of breath, start to sweat, feel lightheaded or dizzy. Some people feel sick, vomit or have persistent indigestion. The symptoms felt during a heart attack do not go away fully with GTN. The longer the artery is blocked before getting to hospital for treatment, the more likely that heart damage will occur. Therefore, if you are having a heart attack it is crucial to phone an ambulance and get to hospital as quickly as possible

> Remember the image of watering the grass? When the water supply is fixed quickly, the grass can recover with no damage. Time is very important! So, if you use your GTN and it doesn't work, phone an ambulance immediately.

There are some common myths and misconceptions about heart attacks (see table 1.2), so learning about these myths will help you understand heart attacks further.

TABLE 1.2   Common Myths and Facts About Heart Attacks

Common myth or misconception	Fact
A heart attack is crushing chest pain (like you may have seen on a poster or on the television).	It may feel that way sometimes but not always. It can be much milder. Remember, if the symptoms don't go away fully with use of GTN, phone for an ambulance.
During a heart attack, the heart stops beating.	Some people confuse the terms heart attack and cardiac arrest. Cardiac arrest occurs when the heart stops beating. Sometimes the heart stops beating during a heart attack, but not always.
Once you have a heart attack, the damage is done.	The sooner you get to hospital for treatment the more likely doctors can save your heart muscle. Heart muscle cells can repair themselves if treatment is started right away to restore blood flow and limit damage.

Treating CHD

Your lifestyle plays a big part in treating CHD and protecting your heart. This aspect of treatment is discussed in detail in the chapters to follow. This section describes medication and possible surgical interventions that can be used to treat CHD.

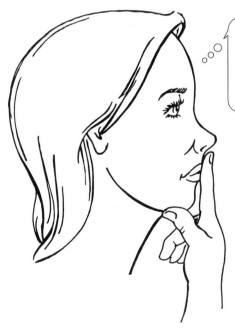

Healthy lifestyle, beta blockers, statins, angiogram, stents, CABG surgery, balloon angioplasty. And I thought aspirin was just a pain killer. What does it all mean?

Medication for Angina or After a Heart Attack

After a heart event, medication plays a big part in your living a long and healthy life. Medications are used to protect your heart, improve your symptoms and improve your quality of life. Despite the fact that medications are effective, people often do not like taking them and do not take them consistently. To increase chances of taking your medications consistently, you must really understand what they do. After having angina or a heart attack you will most likely be on 4 or 5 medications for life. Some of these prescribed medications start off at a low dose and are then increased gradually over the next few months. People often think that increasing the dosage is a bad sign, but it is routine. People are often concerned about side effects of tablets. Sometimes these concerns are from a previous experience or they result from something a friend or neighbour has said or from an article that might tell only one side of the story. If you have concerns, discuss them with your doctor, practice nurse or cardiac rehabilitation professional. Don't let your worries become exaggerated and get the best of you.

A Word About Your Tablets

- Your tablets are an essential part of your treatment.
- If you are worried about side effects, speak to a qualified health professional.
- It is very important that you not stop or change the dosage of your tablets before discussing it with your doctor.

Medications prescribed by your doctor or cardiologist have many positive effects, such as the following:

- They help your heart heal after a heart attack; therefore they help you to have a healthy and active future.
- They reduce the likelihood of a heart attack in the future.
- They thin your blood and reduce the likelihood of blood clots.
- They lower blood pressure, heart rate and cholesterol.
- They reduce your chance of having angina.
- They protect your stent whilst it's healing into place.
- They allow you to exercise more, which helps your heart get stronger and helps you get fitter.
- They reduce the likelihood of CHD plaques bursting. In other words, they stabilise CHD plaques.
- They reduce inflammation in coronary arteries.
- They reduce the problems that can occur if you have an irregular heartbeat.

Table 1.3 lists the most common medications used at the time this book is being published. However, many other medications exist that may be prescribed specifically with you in mind depending on your symptoms, your cardiac history and your CHD risk factors (see chapter 3).

To find out more information about your medication, consult the following websites:

www.patient.co.uk

www.medicines.org.uk/emc

Surgery for CHD

Lifestyle changes and medication are effective ways to improve heart health. However, sometimes surgery is also necessary in order to improve the blood supply to the heart.

What Is an Angiogram?

An angiogram is a test that looks at the coronary arteries and shows where narrowing or blockages exist. The surgeon passes a very narrow tube (a catheter) through an artery in the wrist or the groin. The catheter reaches the coronary arteries and dye is passed through the catheter. At the same time, a scan is being performed; it shows where the dye is *not* flowing properly. In other words, it shows where the arteries are narrowed and how bad the narrowings are.

Percutaneous Coronary Intervention (PCI): Angioplasty and Stent Insertion

Sometimes the angiogram shows that the narrowings in the coronary arteries are not too bad. This means that medication is the best treatment. If the angiogram shows that an artery is badly narrowed or even blocked, the narrowing can be opened using percutaneous coronary intervention (PCI). Opening the artery improves the blood supply to the heart muscle immediately. PCI can be done after a heart attack to reduce heart muscle damage or to reduce the likelihood of angina in the future. It can also be done if angina symptoms are not being controlled well enough with medication and the patient is at risk of having a heart attack in the future. Angioplasty (also known as balloon angioplasty) and stent insertion are types of PCI. Angioplasty is a procedure during which a balloon is passed along the catheter to press back the artery wall and widen the blood vessel again. A stent is a metallic mesh tube that can be inserted to act as a scaffold and hold the artery open (see figure 1.2). Your doctor will decide which type of PCI to use depending on the size of the artery and the nature of the narrowing.

TABLE 1.3 Common Types of Heart Medication and Their Uses

Medications	What they do
Antiplatelet drugs: Aspirin Clopidogrel Prasugrel Ticagrelor	**Reduce blood clotting.** They do this by making some cells in the blood less 'sticky', lowering your chance of having another heart attack in the future. It is likely that you will be on aspirin for life. If you have had a stent it is likely that you will be on both aspirin and clopidogrel, prasugrel or ticagrelor for a period of time that your consultant decides. Clopidogrel, prasugrel and ticagrelor have the added benefit of protecting the stent while it heals into place.
Beta blockers: Atenolol Bisoprolol Carvedilol	**Lower heart rate.** This means that your heart does not have to work as hard. Beta blockers have many complex actions. Having a slower heart rate has many benefits, including prevention of angina attacks, lower blood pressure, and lower risk of having another heart attack.
Angiotensin converting enzyme (ACE) inhibitors: Lisinopril Perindopril Ramipril	**Lower blood pressure and increase the supply of blood and oxygen to the heart.** ACE inhibitors have many complex actions. After a heart attack the heart muscle can be damaged and weakened. ACE inhibitors help the heart muscle to heal and slow down any further weakening of the heart muscle.
Statins: Atorvastatin Fluvastatin Pravastatin Rosuvastatin Simvastatin	**Lower cholesterol and reduce the likelihood of CHD plaques bursting.** Every body has cholesterol in it, but it is impossible to tell how much you have in your body without a blood test. High cholesterol increases your risk of developing CHD. Statins reduce cholesterol levels and therefore reduce the risk of heart attacks.
Nitrates: GTN spray or tablets Isosorbide mononitrate (ISMO)	**Relax the blood vessels round the body and to the heart.** This reduces the workload on the heart and increases the blood flow to the heart. GTN provides rapid relief of angina. It is quick acting and lasts for 20-30 min. ISMO prevents angina and it is long acting.

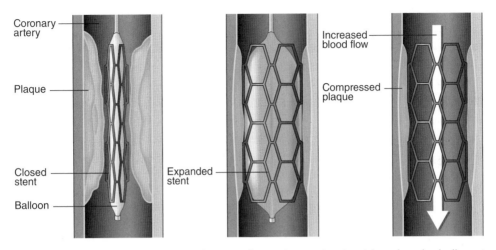

Figure 1.2   Balloon angioplasty involves a collapsed stent that is widened as the balloon is inflated. The catheter is then removed, and the stent keeps the artery open.

What Is Coronary Artery Bypass Graft Surgery (CABG or Bypass Surgery)?

Sometimes the angiogram shows that it is not possible to treat significant narrowings in coronary arteries with balloons and stents. This depends on how many, how bad and which coronary arteries are narrowed. In this case, heart surgery is an option for some people. This surgery is called coronary artery bypass grafting (CABG), or bypass surgery. During bypass surgery, the breastbone is opened (a sternotomy). The narrowed parts of the coronary arteries are then *bypassed* using a graft. This graft is from a blood vessel taken from somewhere else in the body such as a small artery from the chest wall (internal mammary artery), from a vein taken from the leg (saphenous vein) or from an artery from the arm (radial artery). This may sound scary, but don't worry. The body has an amazing ability to compensate once these blood vessels are removed; it can cope without them. The heart surgeon joins one end of the graft to the aorta and attaches the other end below the narrowing in the coronary artery. The heart is then able to receive enough blood flow again.

❤ Remember This

The benefits of medications, balloons, stents and bypass surgery need to be supported by a healthy lifestyle. This book shows you why and how.

After your heart event and treatment, it's really important that you understand how and what you are feeling both physically and emotionally. Understanding these feelings will help you get on the road to a healthy recovery and will help you feel ready to make any changes in your lifestyle that are important to you. Read on to the next chapter to find out more.

What Happens After a Heart Event

People often take their health for granted, so it's only natural that having ill health creates various emotional reactions, including worry and fear. If you have had a heart event, remind yourself that your emotions about the event and its effects on your life are normal. You might be in shock or in denial. You may feel vulnerable and scared. You might be angry with yourself or angry that it has happened to you. You might be forgetful or find it difficult to concentrate. One day you may be positive and hopeful and the next day you may feel exhausted and tearful. You might feel lucky to have a second chance or relieved that you have the opportunity to reassess your life. All these feelings—the ups and the downs—are completely normal.

Your Feelings

I knew there was something wrong; I hadn't felt right for months. At least now I know what's wrong and I can get better. I actually feel relieved.

Gerry, age 50

Once I was home after my heart attack I'd be fine one day—feeling positive and getting on with things—and then I'd be tearful at silly little things, like a hug from my friend or when my neighbour brought me some lovely soup. I felt so grateful and vulnerable at the same time.

Anne, age 52

Often, even after you appear to have coped with the diagnosis, fears can surface. You may feel anxious and a bit depressed, you may have problems sleeping or your confidence may feel shattered. Be patient; many of these feelings gradually fade away as your rehabilitation progresses and you get your confidence back. Going to cardiac rehabilitation, taking part in regular exercise and sharing your feelings with others are helpful in your recovery. Moreover, being with people who are going through the same experiences can be a massive support. And of course, having fun helps, too!

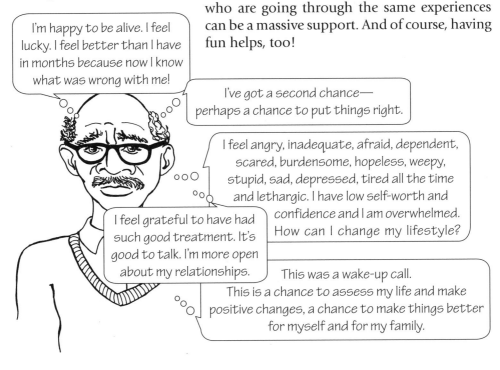

I'm happy to be alive. I feel lucky. I feel better than I have in months because now I know what was wrong with me!

I've got a second chance—perhaps a chance to put things right.

I feel angry, inadequate, afraid, dependent, scared, burdensome, hopeless, weepy, stupid, sad, depressed, tired all the time and lethargic. I have low self-worth and confidence and I am overwhelmed. How can I change my lifestyle?

I feel grateful to have had such good treatment. It's good to talk. I'm more open about my relationships.

This was a wake-up call. This is a chance to assess my life and make positive changes, a chance to make things better for myself and for my family.

At first I found it hard to talk to my wife and children about how I was feeling. I felt I'd let them down and I didn't want to burden them. That's why it was great to speak to the cardiac rehabilitation physiotherapist and to the other people in the exercise class. It felt great to talk when I didn't feel any pressure.

Hanif, age 42

Speaking to other people who had a heart attack and bypass has really helped. It was great to hear people like me saying how they felt. I thought it was only me that felt this way. Now I know I'm not alone.

Henry, age 67

A guy who was finished with the cardiac rehabilitation programme came to speak to us. He was back on his Jet Ski—not that I could ever Jet Ski, but the fact that he is young and had gone back to what he could do before was brilliant. I feel positive about my future again.

John, age 37

However, sometimes these feelings don't fade. There are lots of reasons why you might continue to feel anxious, angry or even depressed after a heart attack. Maybe you're struggling to get over the shock of having a heart attack, maybe it's because of something that happened before your heart event, maybe it's because you feel you have been given confusing information or maybe you have lots of stress in other aspects of your life (family, job, money) and it has become too much for you to cope with. After a heart attack or diagnosis of angina you can have a lot of negative thoughts and wrong ideas about your future that affect your recovery.

However, you must remember that you are not alone. If you are struggling to move forwards with your recovery, then seek help. Speak to those close you or to your doctor, practice nurse or cardiac rehabilitation team. They can help. Or, you can contact the BHF or CHSS (see appendix F). They are recognised experts in providing accurate education and support.

> After my heart attack I felt so low. It went on for weeks, maybe even months. My husband encouraged me to speak to the cardiac rehabilitation staff. They referred me to the psychologist. It really helped; it was not new to them.
>
> Michelle, age 52

After you have a heart event, health professionals ask you to consider making changes such as stop smoking, increase activity and exercise, change your diet, reduce alcohol consumption, be more aware of stress, and take your tablets. All of these changes require you to take control, which is not always easy. People often feel overwhelmed.

> People keep telling me what I *should* be doing. I just don't feel up to the challenge. What am I supposed to do? I have other priorities like making sure my family is OK. And I'm worried about money.
>
> Chris, age 50

Try to get some support from your family and friends. When you're ready, tackle only one thing at a time. Be kind to yourself. Notice your successes. Tackling one healthy behaviour first often helps you be to be able to think about another. This book gives you lots of ideas on how to change aspects of your lifestyle and how to keep them changed.

Heart Attack or a Panic Attack?

After a heart attack you are much more sensitive to any sensation in your body. Feelings that you would have previously ignored become a possible heart attack. Your nervous system is on edge and your sensation is magnified. Stress, anxiety and panic can feel like the symptoms you expect to feel from your heart. These symptoms include your heart racing, chest discomfort or tightness, light-headedness and shortness of breath. Maybe what you're feeling is actually indigestion or a muscle spasm. In time you learn to tell the difference between muscle aches, indigestion, tension, panic and heart symptoms. A technique for easing anxiety is breathing exercises (see chapter 7). If you experience symptoms that you think might be your heart but you're not sure, you must not ignore them. If the symptoms don't go away after a few seconds and a few deep breaths, use your GTN spray or tablet (see chapter 1). If the symptoms are not related to your heart, the GTN will not do you any harm.

> Initially every bout of indigestion was a heart attack and you can become quite paranoid until you learn to tell the difference. You learn ways to relax and calm everything down.
>
> Stephen, age 48

If you are having a lot of these feelings, then please talk to your doctor, practice nurse or cardiac rehabilitation professional. Receiving support as early as possible helps. Relaxation techniques help as well (see chapter 7).

Energy Levels and Stamina

After a heart attack your energy levels can be low for several weeks. This drop in energy occurs for many reasons. You've been in hospital, your body is getting used to some new medication, your body is healing, and you've had a big shock. After balloon angioplasty and stent insertion you might feel absolutely fine, almost as if nothing has happened. However, sometimes you can feel quite tired for a week or so. Even though it's not major surgery, you have had an operation and your body has to heal.

Try not to worry; your energy levels will return to normal, and worrying just makes you more tired.

Daily light exercise and healthy eating will help rebuild your stamina. Take things a little easier for a few weeks, but don't sit about doing nothing. Light exercise helps your body heal, so try to get out for a walk every day. Just keep it at your own easy pace.

Help your body to heal. Go out for a walk, even 10 minutes to begin with, and build it up to 30 minutes.

Twinges in the Chest

Sometimes people feel absolutely nothing after balloon angioplasty or a stent insertion but it is very common for people to feel twinges in the chest. These twinges are normally felt in the left side of the chest. You can often use your finger to point to where you feel it but you can't see anything. The words that people use to describe them are *fleeting, sharp, lasts for a few seconds, niggle* and *funny feeling.* These are not angina symptoms; they are healing pains and can happen for several months. Your body is healing on the inside, and the stent is healing into place. However, you must be careful: If the twinges last longer than a few seconds you must use your GTN.

> After they put my stents in I had this sharp pain in the left side of my chest. It wasn't there all the time; it lasted only a couple of seconds. I had never felt angina before so I didn't know what it would feel like. I was worried. I spoke to my cardiac rehabilitation physiotherapist and she explained that it was healing pains. This really helped and eventually I didn't feel it any more.
>
> John, age 52

Healing pains: Twinges that last a few seconds are not angina. Take a few deep breaths and relax your shoulders; they will go away.

Pain and Bruising

If you have an angiogram, bruising can occur after the procedure. The amount of bruising varies. The arm can be bruised from the wrist to the armpit, the leg can be bruised from the groin to the knee or you may have nearly no bruising. The arm or leg might ache, feel stiff and feel a bit weak. Over the few days after your angiogram the bruising can travel even further down the arm or leg. Don't worry, this is normal. It is not new bruising; it is just the old bruising travelling down with gravity. Sometimes it can take a few weeks but the bruise will eventually go away. If you have pain in the arm or leg, consider taking a simple pain relieving medication (ask at your local pharmacy). Try to use the arm or leg as you would normally rather than favour it. However, if the wound is at the wrist, avoid heavy lifting, pushing or pulling for 7 days. Also avoid excessive pressure on the wrist or groin for 7 days. Make an appointment with your doctor if you have severe pain, redness, warmth or coldness in the arm or leg or if pus develops at the site of the wound. Remember the following:

- Avoid heavy lifting for 7 days after your angiogram.
- Bruising can take a few weeks to go away and often gets worse before it gets better, this is normal.
- The arm or leg can ache for a few weeks, so take a pain reliever such as paracetamol so that you can continue using the arm or leg.
- Don't avoid movement to protect the arm or leg after your angiogram; use the arm or leg normally as soon as possible.

What Happens After CABG and Valve Surgery

In the build-up to your surgery and during your hospital stay, the health professionals involved in your care often refer to a 6- to 12-week recovery period. This time period is the usual range for healing after heart surgery, however, don't expect too much too soon. Full recovery takes time. You will continue to see progress for many months after the surgery.

Heart surgery is a big trauma on your whole body, not just your heart. Thus, the healing process has many aspects.

> After heart surgery, expect full recovery to take 1 year. Make small goals and appreciate the progress you make each week. Don't expect too much too soon; instead, be confident that slowly but surely you will get there.

Changes in Mood

People often have a mixture of feelings after heart surgery, just as they do after a heart attack. You might be weepy or feel your mood is low. Tell your friends and family how you are feeling. They may be feeling it too and you can support each other. Get into a routine each day: Get up, washed and dressed at the same time each day. Set small goals every day. For example, each day add one new activity to do such as walking to the post box or local shop, going for a walk with a friend, reading a book, making a date with a friend to meet at a cafe or park or do some light housework.

> Get into a routine from day one. Get up, washed and dressed at the same time each day. Every day, challenge yourself to do something new.

Energy Level and Stamina

Some people recover more quickly than others. Nevertheless, the first 6 to 12 weeks after heart surgery can be hard work for everyone. Some people are lucky and feel well after the surgery. They feel the benefit very quickly or don't feel that the surgery has affected them much at all. If you were very well before the surgery and not particularly limited by symptoms such as shortness of breath or angina, you might feel much worse after the surgery, which can be frightening. You can't do nearly as much as you could before, which can be frustrating. If you were very unwell before the operation and unable to be active and live your normal life, then your body was already weak and your recovery can be slow.

> For the first 6 or 8 weeks after my heart surgery I felt completely done in—there's no other way to describe it. But it got better. I think I expected too much too soon.
>
> Sheila, age 52

After my heart surgery I felt so exhausted and weak. The operation was such a shock. We had a trip abroad planned later in the year and I felt like I would never be able to do these things again. I thought everything would have to be cancelled—I thought I would have to cancel my life for a long time—and I wondered if I'd ever be the same again. Now, 5 months later and after 12 weeks of cardiac rehabilitation, I've been abroad, I'm fitter than ever and I feel confident again. I honestly can't believe it and my family can't believe it!

Mary, age 72

Shortness of Breath

Feeling more puffed when you do daily activities is very common after surgery but your breathing should not feel uncomfortable. Remember, you were on a breathing machine during the surgery, so your lungs have to recover as well. Also, your stamina is lower and your muscles are weaker, which makes everything you do feel like hard work. This feeling will pass. At the beginning, take your recovery at a gentle but steady pace and have a rest when you need one. Don't sit for long periods doing nothing but worrying; worrying does not help and can even make things worse. Stand up and move around. The little bits of activity are very important.

> After surgery you need to build your stamina. Sitting for longer than 1 hour is too long. Sit less, move more!

Wound Pain and Healing

After surgery the sternal (chest) wound heals in different stages. The surface wound tends to heal very quickly but the bone underneath takes 6 weeks to heal and 12 weeks to really knit together. This means you should only lift light things for the first 6 weeks (1-3lbs or 0.45-1.36kg), like a shopping bag with bread and a small carton of milk, small pots and pans, a half full kettle. Then gradually build up to heavier things over weeks 7 to 12 (5-8lbs or 2.27-3.63kg), like a vacuum cleaner, a light washing basket, a small bucket. And avoid lifting heavy things until after 12 weeks (children, DIY, heavy gardening, heavy washing baskets). **Try to be sensible.** If you have to lift something take two trips, which means you are reducing the weight you are carrying and you are walking more—which is good activity! Don't fill the kettle completely full. Use two small pots instead of one big one. Have two small bags instead of one big bag. Always remember that everyone heals at a different rate, so listen to your body—it will tell you what is right. The pain at the sternal, or breastbone, wound is variable; most people have good and bad days. You can have a few good days and then have a day when you feel particularly stiff and painful. This is normal. You might only need pain relieving medication for a couple of weeks, but you can need them for anywhere up to 12 weeks. This, too, is completely normal. Some people try to avoid taking pain relieving medication even though they are in pain: don't do this. This decision is a mistake. When you are in pain your muscles tense up, you don't move properly and you become stiff, worsening the pain. Also, pain affects the quality of your sleep. You need sleep to help your body to heal and to recover your energy levels. The last pain medication to stop taking are the ones you take at bedtime. Do everything you can to get a good night's sleep because adequate rest is an essential part of your recovery.

♥ A Word About Pain Medication

- Pain causes muscle tension, lack of movement, more pain, lack of sleep and a slower recovery.
- If you are in pain, avoiding pain relieving medication can worsen your condition and inhibit your progress in recovery.
- If you can't sleep because you are in pain, then take pain relieving medication an hour before you go to bed.
- You will have been prescribed pain relieving medication before you were discharged from hospital. Before increasing or reducing your medication it is important to seek individual advice from your doctor, practice nurse or cardiac rehab professional.

Although the sternum is normally firmly healed by 12 weeks after surgery, you can continue to feel aches and pains for many months. The area around the wound can feel tight for many months because scar tissue is tight. Getting back to normal movement is necessary. Movement helps the scar tissue become more flexible and lack of movement allows the scar tissue to become tighter. Numbness across the left breast and around the wound is common and can last for several months. The numbness can become pins and needles as the nerve endings heal. Over time it will fade, but a small area of numbness immediately around the wound can last forever.

If you have had CABG surgery and you have a leg wound, this wound is often the slowest wound to heal, especially the part at the knee or ankle. You may have appointments with your practice nurse for some time after the surgery to dress the wound as it heals. Even whilst the wound is healing you should keep active. Gentle movement actually encourages blood flow and helps the wound to heal. Just as with the chest wound, it's common to have an area of numbness around the leg wound. This numbness is caused by damaged nerve endings around the wound. As the nerve endings heal, you might feel pins and needles; this feeling is normal. The numbness and pins and needles can go on for many months because nerves are the slowest-healing tissues in the body.

Aches, pains and twinges at the chest wound can go on for many months after surgery. Keep active and gradually get back to normal.

Stiffness in the Neck and Shoulders and Poor Posture

When you are recovering from heart surgery, remember the old saying, *Your leg bone's connected to your hip bone and your hip bone's connected to your back bone.* This is true; your sternum, ribs, spine, neck, collar bones, shoulders and all the muscles in between them are connected. Therefore, this whole area can feel stiff and sore, especially when you first wake from sleep. It is important to keep your neck and shoulders moving. It is natural to want to protect your chest wound, but be aware of your posture. Try not to slouch and round your shoulders forwards. This posture can make your chest feel stiffer and the area across your shoulder blades can start to ache.

Keep Moving

- Don't be afraid to move.
- Movement helps healing.
- Gentle movement is the key!

Follow these simple exercises and tips every day, aiming towards the level of movement that was normal for you before surgery:

- Reach for the highest shelf in your kitchen 10 times with both arms at the same time.
- Look round over each shoulder 10 times slowly. Turning to a greater degree to one side than the other is normal.
- Scratch the middle of your back with each hand 10 times. Being able to reach farther up your back with one hand than the other is normal.
- Ask friends and family to tell you if you're slouching because you probably don't notice when you do it.

Poor Appetite

Poor appetite after heart surgery is common for a few reasons. After surgery some people have a horrible taste in their mouth and sometimes things taste odd, even things you used to really enjoy. Also, it's fairly common for people to feel nauseated, bloated and constipated—all normal reactions to the surgery and possibly because of medications such as anaesthetics, antibiotics and pain medication. As a result of poor appetite, people often feel reluctant to eat. It may take 6 to 8 weeks to regain your appetite but these symptoms will improve over time.

> It's weird, after my bypass operation, I'm not enjoying my mugs of tea anymore. They just don't taste the same.
>
> Shelagh, age 63

> Eat small amounts regularly. After surgery your stomach is often the last thing to get back to normal.

If your appetite is poor, try to have frequent small meals and snacks because your body will tolerate small amounts more easily. Try eating something six times a day: breakfast, mid-morning, lunch, mid-afternoon, evening and before bed. Choose appetising foods that you enjoy and are easy to eat such as yogurt, custard, cream rice, soup or a glass of milk. If you have a dry or metallic taste in your mouth try to drink more fluids, suck sweets or mints, chew gum or eat fruit to help cleanse your palate and stimulate saliva. If you feel nauseated cooking smells may be off-putting, so try cold foods such as sandwiches, cheese and biscuits, cold meat and potatoes or breakfast cereals. To avoid constipation, drink plenty of fluids and include foods high in fibre such as wholegrain breads and cereals, and fresh or dried fruits and vegetables. During this time try to eat a variety of foods you enjoy. There is no need to follow a weight-reducing diet or low-fat diet until you have recovered your appetite and strength. Contact your doctor or cardiac rehabilitation team if you are concerned about your appetite or any unintentional weight loss.

Poor Memory and Concentration

It is common for your memory and concentration to be poor for a while. Don't be hard on yourself. Try reading for a short while and then put the paper or book down. Do a crossword or puzzle but take regular breaks.

> Don't be hard on yourself. Again, little and often is the rule of thumb.

Physical Activity After a Heart Event

For the first few weeks after returning home after a heart attack or heart surgery some people are frightened to move and some people feel as though they can do quite a lot. The key is to gradually build up your level of activity. Your body needs a balance of a bit more rest than normal and light physical activity to promote the healing of your heart and your whole body. The following tips are intended to provide general information. If a health professional has given advice specifically for you then please follow this as they know you best.

- **Get into a routine.** From the first day, get up, washed and dressed each day. Don't stay in bed all day; it's bad for your body and mind.
- **Don't sit for long periods.** Stand up and move about every hour or so, walk from room to room or walk up and down the hallway.

- **Use the stairs.** If you could do stairs before your heart event then you will likely be able to do them after. Just take them at a gentle pace; don't push it so that you are breathing heavily, and have a rest if you need one.

- **Listen to your body.** Spend the first few days at home pottering about the house, do some light dusting or wash a few dishes. Some people spend only a day or two indoors and others may need longer. It depends on how you feel. But don't spend any longer than a week indoors before you get out for your first walk. If it's a nice day, sit outside for a while, get some fresh air and take some slow, deep breaths to relax—it's good for you!

- **Go for a walk every day.** Walking is one of the easiest and most natural forms of exercise. Build it up gradually, aiming to do a little bit more each day if you can. Time your walks rather than measuring them by distance. Start with 5 to 10 minutes and then go a little longer each time you go out. Try to keep it on the flat as much as possible for the first 2 weeks. You can't change the roads, so if you get to a hill, just slow your pace down. Everyone is different. Once you're home you can judge for yourself what is suitable for you by your reaction to the previous day's walk. If you feel tired, then don't go so far the next day. If you feel totally exhausted after a walk, you may have walked too far. You have not done yourself any harm, but don't walk as far or as quickly the following day. Over the first 4 weeks try to gradually build your walking up to 30 minutes at a time or break it up into 2 or 3 shorter walks of 15 or 10 minutes each. Remember to enjoy your walking. Vary your route as much as possible so that you don't get bored. If you have a friend with a car, ask them to take you to a different area. If it's a very cold, windy or hot day your heart is working harder, so on days like this don't walk as far or as fast. If the weather is really bad then avoid walking outdoors for the first couple of weeks. Perhaps someone can take you to a supermarket, garden centre, museum or DIY store so that you can go for a walk. Just stay active.

- **Avoid lifting heavy objects** such as shopping bags, vacuum cleaners, laundry, children, suitcases, furniture, garden rubbish and bins. Avoid any exercise that involves pushing, pulling or forcing an object that is stuck or using your arms above shoulder level for long periods of time. If you are recovering from heart surgery then you should not lift anything heavy for 9 weeks whilst your sternum is healing.

- **Don't exercise straight after eating.** This is good advice for everyone, but it's even more important after a heart event. If you exercise after eating then your heart has to work harder. Allow yourself 2 hours after a heavy meal.

- **Get back to work.** Getting back to a working life is vital. It's not just about money; it assists your recovery in every way—mentally, physically, emotionally and socially. Scientific research has shown that people who delay going back to work for too long slow their progress and even go backwards in their recovery. You and your doctor or cardiac rehabilitation professional will decide what is an appropriate amount of time to be off work and if a change is necessary.

After a heart event individual advice is necessary on returning to driving, sport and flying. Therefore, speak to your doctor or cardiac rehabilitation professional about it and contact the Driver and Vehicle Licensing Agency (DVLA) for advice on returning to driving. Go to www.direct.gov.uk or call 00 44 300 790 6801.

Sex After a Heart Event

Getting back to normal in every aspect of your life is essential to your physical and emotional recovery. People are often concerned about returning to their usual sex life after having a heart event. They wonder whether they are fit enough or whether they will have chest pain when they have sex. There is no set amount of time when having sex is allowed again. Sex does not put a special kind of strain on the heart. Think of sex as another form of exercise; it is no more stressful to the heart than other normal daily activities. A general rule is that once you can comfortably climb two short flights of stairs or walk fairly briskly for 20 minutes you can resume a normal sex life. If you are recovering from heart surgery, remember that it takes 12 weeks for the sternum to fully knit together, so consider your position during sex over this time and make sure that you are not holding up your weight through your arms.

It is fairly common for difficulties in having sex to be a problem before the heart event. For some people it is a symptom of the same disease process that causes CHD, which can affect blood flow throughout your body and can therefore cause symptoms in other parts of your body including your sex organs. For some people the difficulties in having sex are caused by the same unhealthy lifestyles that cause heart disease: lack of exercise, smoking, unhealthy diet and not coping with stress. Sometimes the difficulty in having sex may be from a side effect of the medication you are taking. If you are concerned about this, speak to your doctor, practice nurse or cardiac rehabilitation professional. They might be able to suggest changes to your medication to see if it is the problem.

Aside from your physical concerns, returning to having sex after a heart event can be difficult for many other reasons. You and your partner's anxieties can reduce your interest in having sex. This reaction is normal and will pass as you both get your confidence back and your physical health returns.

To avoid misunderstandings or hurt feelings, talk to your partner about your feelings and any difficulty you are having. Don't avoid having sex for longer than you need to; if you put it off for too long, it can become an even bigger pressure. Talk with your partner and be intimate and loving without either of you feeling the pressure of achieving full intercourse. Usually this part of your life returns to normal as your confidence and physical health improve. If you are still having problems after a few months, don't give up. It is an important part of you feeling like yourself again and it's important for your relationship, so speak to your doctor, practice nurse or cardiac rehabilitation professional. Don't be shy; they have heard many people describe the same story and they can help.

> I spoke to my cardiac rehabilitation nurse about the change in our sex life since my heart attack. I was so nervous but I'm glad I did it. It wasn't new to her. She had some good advice and she's going to speak to my doctor. I felt so hopeless before. At least now I feel that things can get better.
>
> Joe, age 51

For more advice, contact the BHF or CHSS advice lines (see appendix F).

Difficulty Sleeping After a Heart Event

As people age they need less sleep and they tend to wake up more during the night. After a heart attack or heart surgery it is fairly common for people to have trouble getting to sleep or staying asleep. Why does this happen? Your sleep pattern was disrupted in hospital and, if you've had surgery, you might feel uncomfortable or in pain when you lie down or turn over. Also, at first when you come out of hospital you might be frightened to go to sleep in case you become ill. This fear should pass as you start to feel more confident again, but the habit of not sleeping has begun. You feel your sleep is not restful and you feel tired and irritable during the day. You may begin to worry about sleep itself; you go to bed exhausted but become wide awake as soon as your head touches the pillow. Try the following quick tips for good sleeping habits:

- Go to bed and get up at the same time every day. This consistency helps to retrain your body's sleep rhythm.
- Take some light exercise early in the evening.
- Do not doze in a chair. Keep sleeping for bedtime.
- Try to slow down in the hour before going to bed. Have a warm bath, listen to music, read a book or watch a light comedy or romantic film.
- Do not consume caffeinated drinks after 6 p.m. Caffeine is a stimulant that exists in tea, coffee, fizzy drinks, some pain medication, energy drinks and cold remedy drinks. Check the labels on packaging and try to cut down your caffeine intake throughout the day.
- If you rely on alcohol as a nightcap to get over to sleep, try to stop this now. It may help you to fall asleep but as the alcohol level in your blood drops, it will wake you up. It will then be harder to get back to sleep again.
- Do not watch television in bed. It keeps your mind awake and means you associate your bed with television rather than sleep.
- If you are awake for more than 20 minutes, try relaxation techniques (see chapter 7) or get up and go into another room.

Some medications can cause you to have very vivid dreams or even nightmares that wake you. If this is your main difficulty, discuss it with your doctor. If your mood is constantly low, you feel hopeless and you usually wake up early for no reason, you may be depressed. Depression can be helped, so speak to your doctor or cardiac rehabilitation professional about your feelings.

How Your Loved Ones Feel After Your Heart Event

You are going through a mixture of feelings and so are those who care for you. It may even seem as if your personality has changed a little, which can be scary for those closest to you. Your family and friends might be worried that you'll not be the same person again.

When Jim came home from hospital I thought things would never be the same. He was so quiet and when he did speak, he was often short with me. I didn't know what he was thinking or feeling. I didn't want to put pressure on him but I needed to be involved.

Lorna, age 52

♥ Share Your Feelings

- As the saying goes, a problem shared is a problem halved.
- Talking is the key; tell each other your worries.
- Involve your family and friends in your recovery; don't think you are a burden.
- Know that you can support each other.

For partners, family and friends, discharge from hospital can be a difficult time. You have been in hospital with numerous health professionals looking after you and now your loved ones think they must take over. They may be desperate to help you but they don't know what to do. Some people, especially those who care, can be overprotective. Although they mean well, it can stifle or slow down your recovery both emotionally and physically. You must be allowed to do little things around the house and at least look after yourself. If someone does everything for you, your self-esteem and confidence can suffer. If you do nothing, eventually you will believe that you can do nothing, your stamina will not improve and eventually you will believe you are weak and need help with simple tasks.

Remember This

- Doing nothing all day makes you fit for doing nothing.
- If you sit in a chair all day, you are only fit to sit a chair.
- You need to build your stamina and confidence by gradually getting back to normal life.

The best way to help someone after a heart event is to support a healthy, active lifestyle. You and your friends and family will benefit from this attitude. Support a healthy lifestyle with loved ones by doing the following:

- Go for walks together.
- Think about little changes you can make to your diet; look for new recipes together.
- Plan to do active things with family and friends.
- If you stopped smoking, use the money you save on cigarettes to plan an outing with family and friends.

If you or your loved ones have concerns and need some advice, speak with a health professional or contact a recognised body of experts, such as the British Heart Foundation or Chest Heart & Stroke Scotland, as listed in appendix F.

Taking Control

You must make changes to your health to protect your coronary arteries (and bypass grafts) in the future. Stents and bypass grafts are not guaranteed to stay unblocked. You can help to look after them by making some healthy choices and taking your medication. Think about the things within your lifestyle that you would like to change. Be active, eat healthfully, don't smoke, keep on top of your stress levels and keep an eye on your blood pressure and cholesterol levels. Read the chapters that follow to help you to make these changes and get some support from your friends and family to live a happy, healthy, long life.

Remember This

A bright future exists for you and your family and friends. You *can* live a happy, healthy and full life after a heart event.

3

Lower Risk Factors to Protect Your Future

CHD risk factors are conditions, habits and behaviours that increase your chance of developing CHD and increase the likelihood that CHD will worsen (see table 3.1). The more CHD risk factors you have, the more likely you are to develop angina, have a heart attack or need heart bypass surgery. Many CHD risk factors are known to exist; some you can control and some you can't.

TABLE 3.1 **Risk Factors for CHD**

CHD risk factors you *cannot* control	CHD risk factors you *can* control
• Family history of angina or heart attack • Age • Sex • Ethnicity	• Smoking • Lack of physical activity • High cholesterol • High blood pressure • Unhealthy diet • Depression • Uncontrolled diabetes • Consuming too much alcohol (see chapter 6) • Overweight and obesity • Not coping with negative feelings and stress

Think about it. You can take control of the majority of CHD risk factors! The odds are in your favour, so don't gamble with your health; take steps to lower your risk.

A Heart MOT—Looking After Your Engine

When thinking about the health of your heart and controlling CHD risk factors, some people find it useful to think of your body like a car and your heart as the engine. To look after your engine it's important that your car has enough fuel, oil and water. As your car gets older it will run more efficiently, more smoothly and will run for longer if it has regular services. Similarly, to look after your heart, your body needs good nutrition and exercise. As you get older, having regular checkups with your doctor or practice nurse helps you to live a long and healthy life. A car and its engine can be damaged by dirty oil, fuel and debris from the road; by being driven badly; working too hard and overheating. Likewise your body and heart can be damaged by smoking, poor diet, lack of exercise, high blood pressure, high cholesterol, high blood sugars, not coping with stress, and drinking too much alcohol. Look after your body and your heart by addressing the CHD risk factors that you can control.

High-risk behaviours for CHD are things people do that can damage the heart and cardiovascular system such as smoking, inactivity, unhealthy diet and not coping with negative feelings and stress. These behaviours are all equally damaging to your heart. Taking control of one of these lifestyle choices can give you the confidence to take control of the others.

> Don't be overwhelmed. Small changes make a big difference.

Reversing some of these behaviours actually can protect the heart (see table 3.2). Heart-protective behaviours reduce many other CHD risk factors. In other words, you can have an effect on several CHD risk factors by changing just one behaviour such as smoking, how active you are, your diet or how you cope with negative feelings and stress.

Healthy living has been proven to lower your risk of CHD and increase your chance of living a long and healthy life. In 2009, a large study of over 23,000 people showed that adhering to four healthy lifestyle factors had a strong impact on the prevention of chronic diseases by 80 percent. Chronic diseases are long-lasting in nature, such as heart disease, diabetes or cancer. Sir Harry Burns (chief medical officer for Scotland in 2009) summarised the findings of this study into a memorable message, which he called 'the magic formula'.

The Magic Formula[1]:

Don't smoke.

Eat 5 portions of fruit and vegetables per day.

Exercise for 3.5 hours per week.

Keep to a healthy weight and shape.*

*Find out what is a healthy weight and shape later on in this chapter

[1]Earl S. Ford et al, The EPIC study, 'Healthy Living is the Best Revenge', 2009, *Archives of Internal Medicine,* Vol 169, No 15, Aug 10/24.

TABLE 3.2   **Effects of Changing Risky Behaviours**

High-risk behaviour for CHD	Heart-protective behaviour	How adopting this healthy behaviour helps to protect your heart
Smoking	Stop smoking.	Stopping smoking helps to reduce blood pressure, artery wall inflammation, and blood clotting.
Sedentary lifestyle, no regular exercise	Be active throughout your everyday life and exercise regularly.	Living an active life and taking regular exercise help to reduce blood pressure, cholesterol, waist circumference, obesity and stress levels; it also helps to reduce and control diabetes.
Poor diet	Eat a healthy, balanced diet.	Eating a healthy diet helps to reduce blood pressure, cholesterol, waist circumference, and obesity; it also helps to reduce and control diabetes.
Not coping with negative feelings and stress (worry, anxiety, anger, irritability, impatience, fear, tension)	Help yourself to cope with negative feelings and stress. Seek support. (see chapter 7).	Coping with stress and negative feelings helps to reduce blood pressure, cholesterol, blood clotting and artery wall inflammation. It makes you more able to change other unhealthy behaviours, for example smoking, unhealthy diet, poor activity level and drinking too much alcohol.
Drinking too much alcohol	Stop drinking alcohol or drink in moderation (see chapter 6 on alcohol).	Avoiding alcohol or only drinking alcohol in moderation can help to reduce blood pressure, waist circumference, triglycerides and anxiety and makes you more able to change other unhealthy behaviours, for example smoking, unhealthy diet, poor activity levels.

These lifestyle changes are not really magic; you can control them. This chapter discusses them in greater detail. Smoking, being inactive and eating an unhealthy diet are all equally damaging to your heart. Taking control of one of these lifestyle choices can give you the confidence to take control of the others.

Stopping Smoking

Stopping smoking is a very important part of your 'Heart MOT'. Tobacco contains thousands of poisons, including nicotine, carbon monoxide, tar, arsenic, cyanide, ammonia, acetone, benzene, formaldehyde and cadmium. When you ask people how smoking damages their health they are likely to say that it causes cancer. In fact, about one third of all cancer deaths are caused by smoking. The scary truth is that 70 percent of the tar inhaled is deposited in the lungs. Smoking can lead to lung cancer, asthma, chronic bronchitis, emphysema, pneumonia, frequent chest infections and a poorer quality of life caused by reduced ability to perform everyday tasks.

People often know that smoking damages their lungs but they don't realise the extent of the damage. Cigarette smoking is linked to 30 percent of all deaths caused by heart disease. Smokers are twice as likely as nonsmokers to have a heart attack. Smokers in their 30s and 40s are five times more likely to have a heart attack than are nonsmokers. When combined with high cholesterol or high blood pressure, the effect of smoking is even more dangerous for the heart. CHD is generally far more severe and extensive in smokers. People who regularly breathe in second hand smoke are 25 percent more likely to develop heart disease.

Smoking causes heart disease in the following ways:

- It makes your blood sticky so that it clots more easily.
- It damages the inner lining of arteries (remember the hosepipe and the grass analogy in chapter 1).
- It produces chemicals that make the heart beat faster and leads to high blood pressure.
- It causes blood vessels to spasm.
- It triggers irregular heartbeats.
- It reduces HDL cholesterol, also referred to as 'good' cholesterol because it transports excess fats away from the arteries and back to the liver to be processed.
- It reduces the amount of oxygen that the blood can carry so less oxygen is available for all your bodily functions. Your body needs oxygen in order to function. If less oxygen is being circulated then your body—and your heart in particular—has to work harder all the time, leading to damaged cells and organs.

Don't Be Disheartened

- One year after stopping smoking, your chance of having a heart attack is lessened by 50 percent.
- There are benefits to stopping smoking no matter what your age or how long you have been smoking.

Benefits of Stopping Smoking

- Your body can heal itself over time.
- Your blood pressure and heart rate return to normal within 30 minutes of having your last cigarette.
- After 48 hours your lungs start to clear out some of the waste materials left by smoking and the decline in lung function and excess risk of lung cancer halts.
- After 2 or 3 days you are able to taste and smell things better and you are able to breathe more easily.
- Your skin and hair become healthier, making you feel and look better.
- Your whole body receives more oxygen, which in turn helps you feel more energetic.
- After 15 years of not smoking your risk of heart attack is the same as for someone who has never smoked.

Put simply, cigarette smoking affects just about every system in your body. Now that you know *why* you should stop smoking, you can focus on *how* to do it successfully (see figure 3.1).

People are more successful in stopping smoking if

- they are determined to stop,
- they get some support, and
- they use nicotine replacement therapy (NRT).

❤ Nicotine Replacement Therapy (NRT)

- Nicotine is addictive. NRT gives you a low dose of a clean form of nicotine and reduces the withdrawal symptoms.
- NRT gives you time to adjust to a life without smoking.
- NRT is available as patches, gum, nasal spray, inhaler, tablets or lozenges.
- NRT is suitable for most people.
- NRT is easy to use and discreet, and some types are available over the counter.

A lot of support is available to help you give up smoking. It's common that people stop smoking after their heart attack and then fall back into the habit at a later date. So, get some help and stay motivated. Speak to your local stop smoking team, cardiac rehabilitation team, pharmacist or practice nurse. Get your family and friends involved and stay motivated. Seek help from legitimate websites and helplines. Here are a few to get you started:

- **www.smokefree.nhs.uk**—Get free support, expert advice and tools including the Quit Kit to help you stop smoking. Watch videos from real quitters on what helped them stop.
- **www.quit.org.uk**—This UK charity helps smokers to stop. This website provides help and advice for smokers, health professionals, employers and teachers.
- **Quitline (www.canstopsmoking.com; tel: 0800 00 22 00)**—Offers access to local support services using your postcode and offers advice on giving up smoking.
- **Smokeline (Tel: 0800 84 84 84)**—This is the UK's national stop smoking helpline and you can call free between 9 a.m. and 9 p.m., 7 days a week.

If you smoke, don't put it off, stop now. You have the resources and it's never too late.

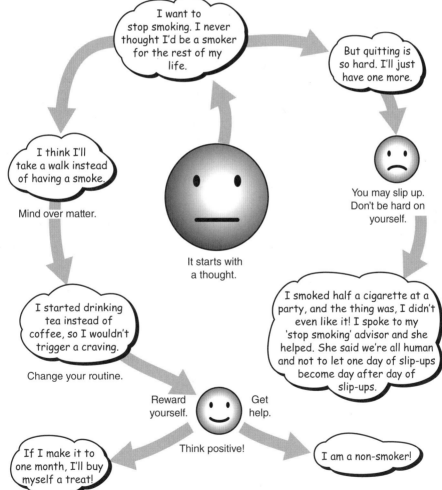

Figure 3.1 The path to quitting smoking has a knock-on effect: It can either lead to success or become a vicious circle.

Living an Active Life and Getting Regular Exercise

Professor Barry Franklin once said that physical inactivity has been called the 'silent killer of our time'.

> Exercise works as nature's medicine to reduce the stress and strain on your heart.

An active life makes people healthy. Scientific research proves it and it simply makes sense. A few generations ago people didn't spend time jogging or going to the gym, but a lot of physical activity was built naturally into their lives. They didn't even have to think about it because they had active jobs and they didn't have cars. But as life has become more and more mechanised with cars and machines, activity during everyday life has declined and so has human health.

Active Habits

To improve your health you need to include active habits in your everyday life. Here are some things you can do to be active without too much thought and planning:

- Walk or cycle to work.
- Climb the stairs.
- Wash the car manually.
- Play with the kids outside.
- Take up active hobbies with friends and family.

Over the years physical activity has often taken a back seat in people's lives. The fact that activity is good for health is not a surprise to most people. But if you ask someone what this means they often struggle to answer. So, think about it this way: There is a minimum amount of activity that everyone should do, regardless of age, to keep the body physically and mentally healthy.

Despite knowing that activity and exercise are good for them, people still have some wrong ideas about activity and exercise.

> As you get older, you have even more reasons to stay regularly active. So families, please encourage your older loved ones; don't take their independence away by being too helpful. Remember, if you sit in a chair all day, you're only fit to sit in a chair!

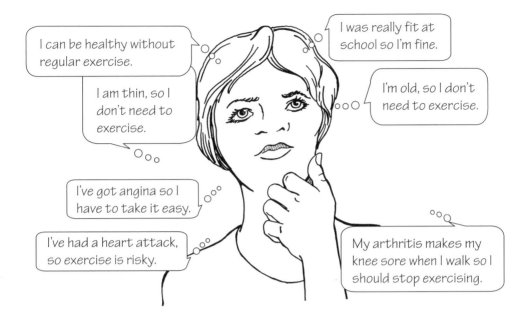

These statements are not based on facts; they are misconceptions and therefore poor excuses for avoiding exercise. Many people think that as they get older, being active is not as important. 'I'm old, I've got a sore knee and my back aches, so I'll just sit here.' Is this you? Everyone needs to do physical activity to be physically and mentally healthy. As you age the type of activity you choose or the intensity with which you do it may change. However, as you age you actually have even more reasons to remain active. Table 3.3 shows many of the benefits of keeping active at any age.

TABLE 3.3   The Benefits of Keeping Active at Any Age

The benefits of activity for everyone	More benefits of keeping active as we age
Regular activity helps to reduce:	Regular activity helps to reduce:
Heart disease	Memory loss and dementia
Type 2 diabetes	Stiff joints and weak muscles
High blood pressure	Restricted movement caused by arthritis
Stroke disease	Falling and breaking bones
Cancer	Struggling with simple daily tasks
Osteoporosis	Dependence on others
Obesity	Being housebound and isolated
Anxiety and depression	
Aches and pains for no reason	

After my heart attack, when I started trying to be more active, all I was thinking about was getting my heart healthy. I started being more active by making sure I sat less and moved more, doing more housework, going for a walk everyday and going to my cardiac rehabilitation exercise classes. I couldn't believe how much it helped the rest of my body. I didn't feel so stiff, my back didn't ache so much anymore, I was able to keep up with my grandchildren a bit better and I felt so much better about myself. I honestly couldn't believe it. I felt like this special secret had been kept from me. I had never really thought about the importance of an active life before. I thought that exercise was for young people. Now I know I was wrong.

Mary, age 83

Getting the Activity You Need

You don't have to go to the gym to have a generally active life. You can make a big difference to your health in simple ways such as by not sitting for long periods and by choosing the active way in your everyday life. The great news is that it does not have to be hard or vigorous exercise for you to get health benefits.

Two Simple Steps to Health

1. Don't sit for long periods; stand up and move every hour.
2. Always choose the active way in your everyday activities (see chapter 5).

Aerobic Exercise

Once you are comfortably achieving enough activity for health (see Two Simple Steps to Health) you should think about working on your aerobic fitness as well. Aerobic exercise makes the heart and lungs use oxygen, and it builds stamina. In other words, aerobic exercise makes you breathe more quickly and works major muscle groups. (Chapter 5 details how to achieve aerobic fitness.) Daily activity helps to protect your heart, but aerobic fitness has an even bigger protective effect: It can help to *reverse* coronary heart disease.

Benefits of Aerobic Fitness

- Reduces the risk of coronary heart disease
- Protects against coronary heart disease
- Can reverse coronary heart disease

People who achieve and maintain aerobic fitness after a heart event significantly improve their chances of living longer. They are 30 percent less likely to have another heart attack or a stroke or die prematurely. So get fit, stay fit, be happy and live longer.

Regular aerobic exercise can reduce, protect against and reverse CHD. It helps arteries to become more responsive when under pressure, which means arteries are less likely to become damaged and clog up with fatty plaque (see chapter 1). In addition, if fatty plaque has started to develop, regular aerobic exercise can stop it from worsening and can even clear out the fatty plaque that is already there.

Regular aerobic exercise makes your heart stronger and more efficient. It improves the heart's ability to transport and use oxygen. If your heart is more efficient, it doesn't have to work so hard during everyday life.

Your muscles become more efficient at using oxygen if you exercise regularly. This reduces the work that the heart and lungs have to do to supply your muscles with oxygen when you exercise. This means that everything you do in your everyday life will feel easier and you will have more energy for simple tasks.

Aerobic exercise helps develop and maintain a good blood supply to your heart. Your body is amazing. If one of your coronary arteries is starting to narrow, regular exercise stimulates new small blood vessels to grow around the narrowed section of the blood vessel. This is called *collateralisation*.

Aerobic exercise helps make the blood less likely to clot and it also increases the amount of 'good' cholesterol in the blood. This is called HDL (high-density lipoprotein) and helps protect the heart by transporting excess fats away from your arteries and back to the liver for processing. Additionally, regular exercise helps to reduce blood pressure as muscle function improves and the whole cardiovascular system becomes more efficient.

Exercise helps to reduce stress, thereby reducing damaging stress hormones in the blood that can injure the artery walls, raise blood pressure, raise heart rate and cholesterol levels and make the blood more likely to clot.

Regular exercise burns calories and helps control weight, which also helps to keep blood pressure down. Exercise builds muscle, which helps to increase metabolism and burn fat. It also improves body shape. People who exercise regularly tend to carry less fat around the abdomen and therefore they have less fat around their major organs, which helps to manage blood pressure and blood sugar levels better and helps to protect the heart. Some people who exercise regularly still carry some extra weight, but being physically active and fit significantly reduces the ill effects of excess weight. If you exercise regularly, the shape around your abdomen, not necessarily your weight, is the important factor. So, don't just use the scales as a measure of your progress. Keep an eye on how your clothes feel around your waist.

Regular exercise can increase feelings of self-respect and confidence. This can make you feel more ready and able to tackle other health changes such as adding healthy choices to your diet and stopping smoking.

Eating a Healthy Diet

A healthy diet contains a balance of fruits and vegetables, carbohydrate (starchy foods such as bread, potatoes and grains) and protein (lean meat, fish, dairy foods and vegetarian alternatives). A healthy diet is low in saturated fat, sugar and salt (see chapter 6). Adopting a healthy diet can protect your heart and helps to reduce your risk of CHD in the following ways:

- It lowers blood pressure.
- It prevents blood clots that can cause heart attacks and strokes.
- It helps to control diabetes; uncontrolled diabetes can lead to damage of blood vessels. This in turn can increase the risk of heart disease, stroke and poor circulation.
- It increases HDL (high-density lipoprotein) cholesterol, also referred to as 'good' cholesterol. Rather than depositing 'bad' cholesterol in the arteries, HDL cholesterol transports excess fats away from your arteries and back to the liver for processing. It reduces LDL (low-density lipoprotein) cholesterol, also referred to as 'bad' cholesterol. LDL cholesterol is carried from the liver to the body's cells. High levels over time can form fatty deposits in the arteries and contribute to heart disease.
- It reduces triglyceride levels. Triglycerides are another type of fat found in the body, which the body stores unused calories for energy. Excess energy from food and alcohol is associated with increased triglycerides. High levels are associated with an increased risk of CHD.
- It helps to keep your body a healthy weight and shape.

Being overweight puts more strain on your heart and all your body organs, including the heart. It can also increase your risk of developing a number of other health conditions such as high blood pressure, type 2 diabetes, stroke and some cancers. If you are overweight, losing just 5 percent of your body weight will improve your health.

Your body shape is even more important when trying to improve your health. Carrying fat around your abdomen (abdominal fat) is a greater health risk than carrying fat around your hips and legs (gluteofemoral fat). People who are apple shaped tend to carry excess fat around the middle. People who are pear shaped carry excess fat around the hips and legs (see figure 3.2). If you are an apple shape, it is even more important that you take action to achieve a healthy weight and shape.

But please don't obsess about it. Some people naturally carry small deposits of fat around the abdomen middle even though they eat healthfully and exercise regularly. The important thing is to live a balanced, healthy lifestyle.

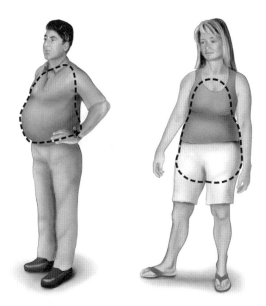

Figure 3.2 Apple and pear shapes. People with apple shapes are more at risk for developing certain diseases.

How to Keep an Eye on Your Weight and Shape

1. Measure your waist circumference. Find your true waist by feeling for the top of your hip bone on one side and moving upwards until you feel the bottom of your ribs. Your waist is in the middle. For most people the waist is level with the navel. Use a tape measure and place it directly on the skin or over a thin layer of clothing to measure around your waist. Make sure the tape measure is snug without squeezing the skin. Use table 3.4 to see if you are at a higher risk of health problems.

2. To check how healthy your weight is for your height, use figure 3.3 by locating your height on the chart and drawing a line across until you find your exact weight.

TABLE 3.4 **Waist Measurement and Risk of CHD**

Waist measurement	Increased risk	High risk
Men	94-102 cm (37-40 inches)	Larger than 102 cm (40 inches)
Women	80-88 cm (31.5-34.5 inches)	Larger than 88 cm (34.5 inches)

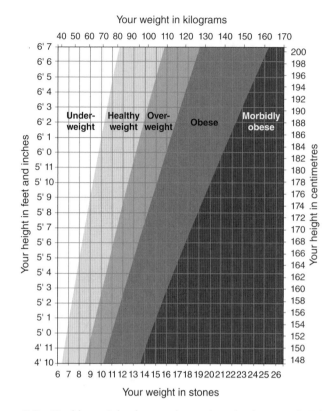

Figure 3.3   Healthy weight chart to determine whether your height and weight correspond to a healthy size.

Coping With Negative Feelings and Stress

In years gone by, medicine focused on physical health only, but now scientists know that emotions, thoughts and feelings affect how well the body functions. A positive mental attitude is now accepted as important in recovering from any health problem and living a healthy life. This doesn't mean that your thoughts must be positive all the time. It's normal to feel sad, angry, scared, stressed or overwhelmed at times. It's important that you acknowledge how you are feeling, get support and move forwards in your recovery emotionally and physically. It's about getting involved in healing your body, increasing your resilience by being optimistic and believing in a positive future.

> You can't detach your body from your mind. Being happy and positive and doing things to help you feel in control affect your physical health.

When you feel worried, tense, scared, angry or stressed, it's usually because a negative thought has increased the amount of stress hormones in your body (adrenaline and cortisol). A rise in adrenaline increases heart rate, blood pressure, cholesterol, artery wall inflammation and blood clotting. When you're stressed, your muscles tense and your breathing becomes shallow and rapid. This isn't bad or danger-ous; in fact, it's completely normal and happens to everyone. The only problem is that it doesn't feel good, and if you have recently had a heart attack or have a lot of worrying and stressful things happening in your life, these negative feelings and high adrenaline levels can be persistent and can last a long time, which can affect your recovery and your future health.

Too much negativity and not coping well with stress affect behaviour. People who are always wor-ried, angry or tense and people who are not coping well with stress tend to reach for the unhealthy behaviour that they think will give them comfort such as cigarettes, high-fat foods, alcohol or inac-

> Think positively and realistically. Do things regularly to relax. Help yourself to stick with a healthy lifestyle.

tivity. Therefore, for the health of your heart and for your general health, try to stop negative feelings from becoming overwhelming and regularly make time for the things that help you to relax (see chapter 7).

Table 3.5 has some common negative and positive thoughts that can occur after having a heart event. Read them and pay attention to how they make you feel. Negative thoughts are in the back of your mind all the time. When you're worried, stressed, afraid or irritable, the negative thoughts are more prominent. And the vicious cycle continues: negative thought, adrenaline, negative thought, adrenaline.

Try to be aware of your negative thoughts and change your focus to being more positive. Switch the adrenaline off and help your recovery and your future health. Read the positive thoughts in table 3.5 regularly to keep you on track and make time for the things that help you to relax (see chapter 7).

> You can save yourself a lot of worry by getting the facts right and planting positive thoughts firmly into your head. So, consider your thoughts in the following ways;
>
> - Are you having lots of negative thoughts?
> - Are you sure your thoughts about your health and your future are accurate?
> - Do you have unanswered questions?
> - Do you need to discuss your thoughts and questions with a health pro-fessional so you can understand and move forwards with a healthier, happier future?

This chapter has presented the unhealthy lifestyle choices that can lead to CHD. This information is a lot to think about and may seem overwhelming at first. However, the following chapters provide straightforward information to help you increase your knowledge and build your confidence so that you can adopt a healthy lifestyle in a way that works for you—one step at a time.

TABLE 3.5 Challenging Your Thinking for a Healthy Recovery

Negative thoughts		Positive thoughts
I'll never be the same; I'm finished.	→→→	Most people make a full recovery after a heart attack. I am getting stronger all the time.
My heart is weak.	→→→	My heart is the toughest muscle in my whole body. My heart is amazing; it is healing itself.
I'm so tired; my heart must be really bad!	→→→	It's normal to feel tired for a while after a heart attack.
Some days I feel so tired; it must be my heart.	→→→	Everyone has days when they feel tired. This is not to do with my heart; it's normal.
If I work too hard I'll have a heart attack.	→→→	Ordinary hard work will not cause a heart attack.
I'll never work again.	→→→	Most people get back to work after a heart attack.
I'm feeling a bit puffed, I'd better rest; I'm weak.	→→→	Exercise is supposed to make you breathe faster and make you sweat sometimes. I'm strong!
I've got no chance of stopping smoking.	→→→	One day at a time. I'm doing really well!
I feel niggles and flutters in my chest. I'm going to have a heart attack.	→→→	Niggles and flutters in the chest lasting for a few seconds are normal and are often from muscular tension.
This exercise feels so hard today; it must be my heart.	→→→	We all have days when exercise feels like really hard work and then days when it feels much easier; this is normal.

4

Monitor Your Activity

One of the first questions that people ask when they start to become active after a heart event is *How do I know if I'm doing too much?* Then, after a couple of months in a cardiac rehabilitation programme, the question often becomes *When I'm exercising, how do I know if I'm working hard enough?*

The mind is an excellent judge of how much work the body is doing. How physical activity feels, tells you the intensity of the exercise; in other words, it indicates how hard you are working. To get the most healthy heart benefits from exercise you need to get the intensity right. Exercising at the proper intensity allows you to be active frequently for the right amount of time each week, in a way that is enjoyable and beneficial. Listening to your body comes more easily to some people than to others. People who are generally competitive, high achieving and impatient often find it difficult to listen to their bodies. On the other hand, people who feel anxious or fearful can be very sensitive to sensations of exertion. It is therefore important for you to spend time learning how to listen to your body. This chapter begins to teach you these skills.

> Spend time learning how to listen to your body.

Normal Sensations of Exercise

The best way to know how hard you are working is to learn to listen to your body and get to know the normal sensations of exertion. Normally when you exert yourself you feel warm, breathe deeper, and feel the muscles working.

People have many misconceptions or 'wrong ideas' about how exercise should feel. Some of these misconceptions are discussed next.

- **I feel tired, so I've done too much.** Muscle fatigue is normal and good. If you feel muscle fatigue when you exercise, then your muscles will get stronger and your daily life activities will feel easier. However, if it takes more than 3 days for your muscles to get back to a feeling of no aches or fatigue, then this is a sign you have overdone it.

- **No pain, no gain. I'm totally knackered. I've done enough.** This person is exercising too hard or too fast, which can lead to injury or exhaustion.
- **I need to sweat buckets to get benefit from exercise.** Sweating is healthy and allows your body to cool down, but sweating profusely does not mean you are getting more benefit from the exercise. Many factors affect how much you sweat: When you are fit, your body is tuned in to exercise and starts to sweat more readily. Your body also sweats more in hot or humid climates, if you carry more body fat and if you are unwell. (Don't exercise when you are unwell.) So, don't focus on how much you sweat, but always remember to have frequent drinks of water whilst you exercise to replenish fluids.

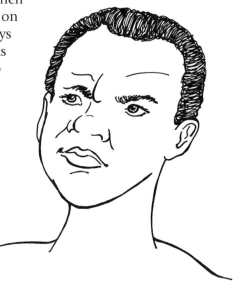

- **I'm hating it, so it must be good for me.** If you hate the type of exercise you are doing, it's very unlikely that you will keep going back for more. If you want to improve your chances of staying regularly active, you must choose a type of exercise that you find challenging but comfortable and fun!

Listening to Your Body

A good way to tune in to how your body feels during exercise is to use a scale that helps you to rate your level of exertion, or effort. The exertion scale is represented in table 4.1 and at the end of appendix E. Please copy or cut it out of the book for reference whilst reading this chapter. The exertion scale method is very reliable; it is used extensively in cardiac rehabilitation programmes. When you tune in to your body whilst you exercise and relate how you feel to the exertion scale, you can become independent, safe and effective at monitoring your levels of exertion. This is not just in terms of structured exercise but in whatever physical activity you perform in your daily life such as gardening, washing the car, housework or climbing the stairs.

TABLE 4.1   **The Exertion Scale—Listen to Your Body**

	How much exertion?	How does it feel in your muscles and breathing?	The talk test
0	Complete rest	Relaxed breathing, relaxed muscles (sitting still)	You can sing and whistle whilst exerting yourself.
1	Minimum effort	Normal breathing, no muscle strain	
2	Extremely mild effort	Just aware of breathing more deeply, aware of very slight muscle strain	
3	Somewhat mild effort		
4	Mild effort	Breathing more deeply, muscles lightly strained	You can talk comfortably whilst exerting yourself.
5	Medium effort	Breathing deeply, definite muscle strain but comfortable, able to continue	
6	Fairly strenuous effort		
7	Strenuous effort	Breathing really deeply, muscles very strained, feeling like you would like to slow down	You are struggling to talk in sentences whilst exerting yourself, gasping for breath.
8	Very strenuous effort		
9	Extremely strenuous effort	The hardest effort you have ever experienced; muscles and breathing are pushed to a very high level	
10	Maximum exertion	The maximal exertion that could possibly be achieved; most people will never experience this	

To use the exertion scale, you must think about the normal sensations of exertion and rate the intensity of those sensations in your body **whilst you are exercising**:

- **Breathing depth and rate**—Ask yourself, 'How puffed am I? How heavily am I breathing? How deeply am I breathing? Can I still talk comfortably whilst exercising?'

- **Muscle sensations**—Ask yourself, 'Are my muscles feeling ache or strain that could lead them to become tired? Do I feel that I am working? Am I comfortable?

- **Body temperature**—You should always feel warm when you exercise, but some people sweat more than others. This depends on your personal makeup and on the environment.

Knowing How Hard You Are Working

When using the exertion scale, first determine how much strain you feel in your muscles and in your breathing. Then look on the scale to the words that best describe these sensations. You will naturally arrive at the number on the scale that corresponds with your effort.

Alan is out for a cycle. He says, 'I feel comfortable but I definitely feel that I am working. I'm breathing harder but I can still talk in sentences. My muscles feel under a bit of strain but I can still do more. I'm definitely warm but it's cool today, so I'm sweating only a little bit. I feel great; I'm having fun. This feels like 6 on the exertion scale.' Alan is exercising at the right intensity to gain health and fitness. This intensity is safe for everyone.

Jim is working out in the gym. 'I'm breathing more deeply but I'm not gasping. My muscles are getting tired but I'm comfortable. I'm having fun! I feel that this exercise is medium exertion, or 5 on the exertion scale.' Jim is exercising at an intensity where he will develop aerobic fitness and help to keep his heart healthy.

Anne is out for a walk. She says, 'I'm not really breathing any more heavily; my muscles are working but it feels very light. I feel that this exercise is very light, or 2 on the exertion scale.' The intensity of Anne's exercise is too low to be completely effective. She needs to increase the effort. She could do this by picking up her pace or by choosing a route where she climbs some hills.

Margaret is at an exercise class. She says, 'I'm exhausted; I need to have a rest. I'm gasping for breath and I can't even talk in sentences without puffing halfway through. This is not fun! I feel that this is very hard, or 8 on the exertion scale.' Margaret needs to slow down a little. At this intensity she is more likely to injure herself or not go back to the exercise class because it isn't fun.

How Hard Am I Working?

Try this when you are exercising. Ask yourself how hard you are working and consider these three questions:

- *How much strain do I feel in my muscles? Am I challenged but comfortable?*
- *Can I still talk in sentences without puffing halfway through?*
- *Am I having fun?*

Whilst you are exercising, try to keep the exertion scale in your mind and listen to your body. Think about how hard you are finding the exercise. How exerted do you feel? To keep healthy with exercise you should feel warm, you should be breathing deeply but always be able to speak in sentences and the muscles you are working should feel strained but not painful. In other words, you should feel challenged but comfortable, and most of all you should have fun.

5

How to Be Active and Fit

You know now that being active benefits the whole body and should be a part of everyone's daily life, regardless of age or medical history. You can help to protect the health of your friends and family by encouraging them to be active, too. Involving your friends and family makes it easier for you to get going and keep going. You understand why you should be active and how it should feel after a heart event. Now you must understand what to do and how to do it. A lot of information exists about exercise and plenty of people want to tell you what to do. It can get confusing, which can put you off. To make it clearer, you can follow three steps, which are listed in the activity pyramid in figure 5.1.

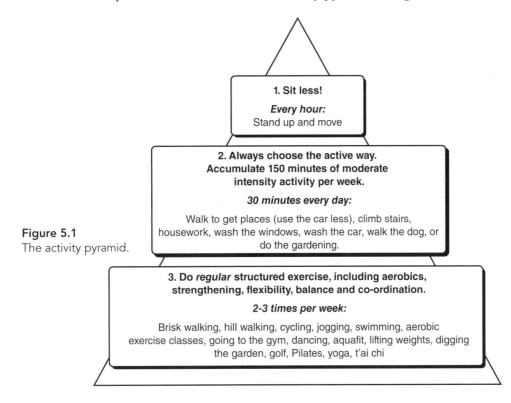

1. Sit less!

Every hour:
Stand up and move

**2. Always choose the active way.
Accumulate 150 minutes of moderate
intensity activity per week.**

30 minutes every day:

Walk to get places (use the car less), climb stairs,
housework, wash the windows, wash the car, walk the dog, or
do the gardening.

Figure 5.1
The activity pyramid.

**3. Do *regular* structured exercise, including aerobics,
strengthening, flexibility, balance and co-ordination.**

2-3 times per week:

Brisk walking, hill walking, cycling, jogging, swimming, aerobic
exercise classes, going to the gym, dancing, aquafit, lifting weights, digging
the garden, golf, Pilates, yoga, t'ai chi

Some people may find it difficult to achieve all three steps of the activity pyramid because of ill health or physical restrictions. Increasing your activity levels even slightly will improve your general stamina, strength, flexibility and balance. Any improvements in any of these areas are beneficial. Simply 'sit less and move more', aiming to do as much as you can. You may be able to do more than the three steps of the activity pyramid, and that's great too. The more, the better.

Sit Less

The top of the activity pyramid encourages you to sit less. Many people are sedentary (sitting or lying) for more than 7 hours a day (not including sleeping). This statistic is even worse for older people, many of whom can sit for longer than 11 hours a day. Generally sedentary time increases with age. The longer the sedentary period without standing up, the worse it is for your health. What does 'bad for your health' mean? Well, spending your life with long periods of sitting makes you much more likely to develop heart disease, obesity, diabetes and some cancers. It therefore shortens life expectancy. Studies of people in the United Kingdom and the United States have found that many people sit for 4 to 5 hours without standing at all. Much of the sitting time is spent watching television, using computers, driving, talking on the phone, reading or listening to music. Aim to break up this pattern of behaviour. Just stand up and move, walk about a bit or climb the stairs. In other words, just *move*.

> **Prolonged sitting is bad for your health. Sit less, stand up and move around frequently. Move every hour.**
>
> *To try to help me to stop eating so much chocolate, someone said I should think of more than 2 chocolates as an overdose of chocolate, so I was thinking, is sitting for more than an hour an overdose of sitting?*
>
> George, age 72
>
> Although this patient's statement is funny, the answer is actually yes. Spending your life sitting for long periods is bad for your health and can shorten our life. Avoid overdosing on sitting. Get up and move.

To increase your chances of success, make yourself a plan for sitting less and moving more. Think of all the times when you sit for longer than 1 hour and think of ways to break the pattern, such as the following:

- When watching television, get up and move when there are adverts or when each programme ends. Walk to the kitchen, get a glass of water or wash a few dishes.

- Put a brightly coloured sticker on your computer or set an alarm to remind you to get up and walk for a couple of minutes every hour.
- When driving long distances, stop your car in a lay-by or a quiet road and walk round the car 5 times.
- On a train, stand for the last few stops so that you are not sitting for the whole journey.
- In a plane journey, get up and walk to the back of plane every hour if it is safe to do so.

Now, make your plan. Write your own list of ideas and stick it to your telly, computer, fridge or notice board. It might feel silly, but visual reminders really work. Appendix A, Templates for Helping You Plan, provides forms for you to cut out or print out and use. Make a commitment and share it with someone who will support you to do what you want to do. Get a family member or friend to witness it. It's much more fun to get healthy when you and your loved ones support each other.

> Remember that small changes make a big difference!

Always Choose the Active Way

The middle of the activity pyramid encourages you to improve your health by building activity into your daily routine. Like we mentioned in chapter 3, people didn't have to think consciously about being active in the days when they had active jobs and fewer cars. They just did it as part of their lives. However, in modern times you must make a conscious choice to have an active life.

> Have you been sitting reading this book for longer than an hour? Get up and move!

Having an active life means you are much less likely to have heart disease, diabetes, high blood pressure, stroke, cancer, osteoporosis, obesity, anxiety, depression, and aches and pains for no reason. If you remain active as you age, you are much less likely to have memory loss and dementia, stiff joints and weak muscles, and falls and broken bones. You are also much less likely to be restricted by arthritis, dependent on others, housebound and isolated. You won't be as likely to struggle with simple daily tasks.

For Better Health

- Accumulate at least 150 minutes (2.5 hours) of moderate-intensity activity each week. A good way of doing this is 30 minutes of activity per day, preferably every day.
- Do at least 10 minutes of activity at a time.
- Remember that more than 150 minutes per week is even better.

You don't have to do everything all at once; thinking about 150 minutes at a time can seem overwhelming and even impossible. Start with little bits and build it up; make it possible for yourself. Try doing 15 stairs, 4 times a day. You would climb Ben Nevis in a month!

After my heart attack I started to do more gardening. Now I am a member of the local gardening club and have won prizes for my begonias. I never thought I'd love it so much.

Eck, age 55

You can build activity into your day by breaking some bad habits and getting back some good habits. Do any of the following statements sound familiar to you?

- I used to walk to the newsagent's daily, but the bad weather stopped me and I never got back into it. I got used to just jumping in the car.
- I used to go for a walk in my lunch break with my friend, but he changed jobs and I gave up my walk.
- I used to climb one flight of stairs when I lived on the first floor, but now I live on the tenth floor so I just take the lift.
- I used to walk or cycle to work, but we moved farther away. So I drive to work and park in the car park out the back.
- I used to do all my own housework, but I had a heart attack and my daughter started doing it for me. I think I could do it now but I don't feel confident and I like my daughter coming round.
- I used to get the bus into town to go shopping, but after I had my heart bypass I started taking a taxi. I think I could use the bus again but I'm not sure.

- I used to take my dog for a walk, but now I just go to the park and let her run round.

Table 5.1 shows an example of an active day. This day might look like a lot, but your active days can begin with some activity and then build up to more activity. Notice that the activity is spread throughout the day.

TABLE 5.1   **A Very Active Day**

9 a.m.	Walked dog for 10 minutes
10:30 a.m.	Washed car, cut grass and swept path for 30 minutes
Noon	Took bus to town, got off 2 stops early, walked the last bit
12:30 p.m.	Walked up and down 2 flights of stairs in store when shopping
2 p.m.	Took bus back home, got off 2 stop early and walked rest of way
3 p.m.	Took dog out again 20 minutes
8 p.m.	Took dog out for evening walk 10 minutes

Once you choose to live an active day, these statements may sound more familiar to you:

- If it's going to be a short walk, I'll make a point of not taking the car. It's surprising how far I can get in 10 minutes.
- My daughter came with me on the bus a few times and now I can do it by myself. I feel more like myself again. Jean and I are going to get the bus to the coast on Friday. I can't wait!
- At least twice a week I take the dog to various places for a longer walk. She loves it and so do I. I think I'll do it more often now.
- I always try to climb at least one flight of stairs, then I get the lift if I have to.
- I go for a 10-minute walk in my lunch break. I love the peace and quiet and I feel less tense when I come back.
- I take the train to work so I've got a 20-minute walk either side. It sets me up for the day and I get home feeling less hassled.
- I park my car a 10-minute walk away from work.
- I always try to get off the bus a stop early and walk for 10 minutes.
- I do all my own housework now. And because she's not cleaning for me anymore, my daughter and I spend time going for walks instead.
- I wash my car by hand. I actually do a better job than the machine.
- I wash my own windows.
- I can't do all the heavy gardening but I do what I can and I love it!

Now, write your own list and stick it somewhere you'll see it at the start of each day. The form in appendix A, Planning Your Activity: Accumulate 30 Minutes, will help you get started. You can cut it out or print it out, then fill it out for yourself. Remember to get some support. If you have children or grandchildren, ask them to sign it; they are great motivators. Get them to join in. They can make their own list. Encourage their activity and make it fun!

Perform Regular Structured Exercise

The bottom of the activity pyramid encourages you to perform structured activity to develop fitness. A question that people who have had ill heart health often ask is *What is the best form of structured exercise to do?* The answer is *Build up gradually, keep it safe, and make it balanced and fun.*

Build Up Gradually

If you are taking up activity and exercise for the first time or you are rediscovering it after a period of inactivity, you should build it up gradually. Start with light activities such as gardening or walking. Build more activity into your daily life first, accumulating shorter bouts of 10 to 15 minutes, then progress to longer structured exercise sessions. Once you are ready to start your structured exercise sessions, start gently; don't go too fast or too hard. Always remember how it should feel (see chapter 4).

Keep It Safe

The following safety points are especially important to follow when exercising after a heart event.

- Always warm up and cool down; start slowly and finish slowly.
- Don't exercise on an empty stomach. Eat a light snack 1 hour before you exercise.
- Don't exercise on a full stomach. Always give your body a chance to digest food before giving it more work to do. Allow 1 hour after a light meal and 2 hours after a large meal.
- Drink water during exercise to keep well hydrated.
- Don't exercise if you have an infection or are on a short course of antibiotics. At this time your body is working hard enough to fight off the bug, so don't challenge it even more with exercise. If you feel up to it, just go out for a gentle walk to get some fresh air. (Some people are on longer-term antibiotics for various reasons. If this is the case, seek some advice from your doctor, practice nurse or cardiac rehab professional).
- Don't exercise the day after drinking too much alcohol (more than 3-4 units for men and 2-3 units for women); in this situation your body is

working harder when trying to exercise while coping with the effects of alcohol. Just go out for a gentle walk.

- When you start exercising again after a break, especially if you have been unwell, don't push too hard; start off with light exercise. Choose a type of exercise that you find easy and enjoyable, such as walking.

- Pay attention to the weather. If you normally exercise outside (walking, hill walking, cycling) be aware that your body is working harder in extremes of weather (very hot, very cold or very windy). On days like this, don't go so hard or so far and give your body longer to warm up and cool down.

- If you have had a heart attack or have angina, then you will have a GTN spray or tablets. Always make sure you carry your medication, even if you have not needed it for years. If you need it, you need it *now* and not when you get home.

- If you like to exercise by yourself sometimes, then it's a good idea to tell someone where you are going and how long you'll be.

It can be a hassle to carry extra things when you go out and it's so easy to forget small things. So, plan ahead to ensure your safety: Always have a few GTN sprays and put one in each bag or coat. If you need it, you need it *now*, not when you get home.

Make It Balanced and Fun

A balanced exercise programme involves two or three bouts per week that improve aerobic fitness, strength, flexibility, balance and coordination. Balancing various types of exercise can benefit you in many ways. See the following types of exercise and their benefits:

- An aerobic fitness class, hill walking and a gym session—these types of exercise build aerobic fitness, strength, and balance and coordination.
- T'ai chi, yoga and Pilates—these types of exercise build strength, flexibility, and balance and coordination.

It may feel overwhelming to create a balanced programme for yourself. Examples of how to accomplish this are discussed later in the chapter.

Aerobic Exercise

Aerobic exercise means activity that builds stamina and makes your heart and lungs use oxygen. Aerobic exercise involves continuous, rhythmic movement of your large muscle groups over a sufficient period of time. Remember, your heart benefits most from aerobic fitness. Table 5.2 lists other benefits, too.

TABLE 5.2   Exercise to Improve Aerobic Fitness

Benefits of regular aerobic exercise	Types of exercise for aerobic fitness
<ul><li>Strengthens your heart</li><li>Boosts your good cholesterol</li><li>Helps to lower your blood pressure and heart rate (so your heart isn't working so hard)</li><li>Makes your blood less likely to clot</li><li>Helps to clear out clogged arteries and helps arteries become more able to cope with pressure</li><li>Helps to reduce fat around your waist and belly</li><li>Helps with weight loss</li><li>Helps to reduce your risk of developing diabetes</li><li>Helps to control diabetes</li><li>Makes you feel good</li><li>Reduces stress and tension, helps you to relax</li><li>Helps improve anxiety and depression</li><li>Helps to keep your muscles and bones strong</li><li>Improves your self-esteem</li><li>Keeps your joints mobile</li><li>Helps to prevent ill health (cancer, stroke, dementia)</li><li>Increases your life expectancy</li></ul>	<ul><li>Brisk walking, hill walking, rambling</li><li>Dancing, such as Scottish country dancing and ballroom dancing</li><li>Cycling</li><li>Swimming</li><li>Aerobic gym equipment such as treadmill, stair stepper, rowing machine or exercise bike</li><li>Aerobic circuit classes</li><li>Stair stepping</li></ul>

A Word About Diabetes

- CHD is generally more severe in people with diabetes. It is therefore even more important to take control of other CHD risk factors such as smoking, diet, exercise, cholesterol, blood pressure, and stress management.

- Physical activity is proven to control blood sugar levels and improves how the body uses insulin.

- Physical activity is known to be a key element in the prevention and management of type 2 diabetes.

- Physical activity and modest weight loss have been shown to lower the risk of type 2 diabetes by 58 percent.

- If you have diabetes, it is important that you ask for some advice from your doctor or nurse before undertaking new exercise.

For more information and support see www.diabetes.org.uk

To be classified as aerobic, the exercise must meet the FITT principles: *frequency, intensity, time and type*. Furthermore, if you are to stay motivated and stick with an exercise regimen, exercise needs to be fun. So, once you add *enjoyment*, it becomes the FITTE principle, as shown in table 5.3.

TABLE 5.3   **FITTE Principles**

Principle	Explanation
Frequency—how much?	Perform aerobic exercise at least 2 times per week.
Intensity—how hard?	The exercise should make you breathe more deeply and feel warm. Your muscles should feel strained but not exhausted.
Time—how long?	Each session should last 45 minutes to 1 hour. This is made up of 1. a 15-minute warm-up, 2. 20- to 35-minute overload, exertion level 4-6 (see chapter 4; increase time as you get fitter) and 3. a 10-minute cool-down.
Type—what to do?	Try brisk walking, cycling, swimming, a gym programme, aerobic exercise class or dancing.
Enjoyment—keeps us motivated.	It must be fun!

Performing aerobic exercise two or three times per week is a sufficient frequency to develop fitness and achieve all the heart benefits that comes with aerobic fitness. Chapter 4 discussed intensity and how exercise should feel. Table 5.2 provides examples of various types of aerobic exercise.

Another important point to think about is how continuous is your aerobic exercise? You might have noticed that table 5.2 doesn't contain activities such as golf and bowling. Golf and bowling are great activities but they are not continuously aerobic. If you enjoy exercise that is less continuous, then try to incorporate something else from table 5.2 as well to gain more healthy heart benefits.

Another aspect of the FITTE principle is time. For exercise to be safe it is important to gradually increase (warm up) and gradually decrease (cool down) the heart rate and blood pressure and therefore the workload on the heart. When you exercise, the heart needs more oxygen-filled blood and it takes time for blood flow to increase to the heart. These processes are even more important as people age and in people with CHD. If you warm up too quickly you are more at risk of experiencing angina.

Start slowly and finish slowly. Keep it safe!

If you cool down too quickly you are more at risk of an irregular heartbeat, especially if you are exercising quite hard. If you cool down too quickly, you are also more at risk of a sudden drop in blood pressure, which will make you feel lightheaded. In addition, your muscles, tendons, ligaments and joints need time to warm up and move freely, and to cool down gradually without stiffening up. A safe and effective warm-up takes about 15 minutes. A safe and effective cool-down takes about 10 minutes.

Strengthening Exercise

Remember, to keep your heart healthy, strengthening exercise should be undertaken **in addition to regular aerobic exercise.**

There are lots of benefits from regularly performing strengthening exercise and lots of different ways to do it (see table 5.4).

After the age of 40, the natural progression of the human body is to lose muscle bulk. As they get older people often complain of bad balance. Feeling unsteady and unsafe affects confidence and independence. Commonly the bad balance is actually due to weak muscles. Therefore, as you get older, it's even more important to begin or continue exercising to maintain and build strength, to increase your confidence and to keep you independent.

For years, people with heart disease were advised to stay away from strengthening exercise. However, it has now been proven that if done the right way, it is completely safe and beneficial. Nevertheless, you must get some advice from a trained professional.

TABLE 5.4   **Exercise to Improve Strength**

Benefits of strength exercise	Types of exercise for strength
• It helps to maintain strong muscles and bones. • It reduces your heart rate and blood pressure, thereby reducing the strain on your heart when you are performing daily manual jobs such as carrying groceries or lifting heavy objects. • It raises your metabolic rate, thereby helping you to stay leaner. • Stronger, larger muscles burn more calories, helping to reduce body fat. • It increases our energy and stamina. If you are strong, everything you have to do in your daily life feels easier; if you are weak, everything is an effort and feels like hard work. • It helps you to have good balance.	• Climbing stairs • Walking uphill • T'ai chi • Pilates • Yoga • Lifting weights (dumbbells or free weights, squats, sit-ups, press-ups, weight machines).

When you perform strengthening exercises, remember the following guidelines to keep you safe:

Because you lose muscle bulk as you get older, strengthening exercise is even more important as you age.

- Don't hold your breath. Practice slow, relaxed breathing.
- If you are lifting a weight, breathe out as you lift it and breathe in as you lower it back down again.
- Practice good posture. Pull in your tummy muscles and stand up tall.
- Don't lock your joints; rather than straighten them completely, keep them slightly bent as you use your muscles.
- Always lift and lower the weight smoothly and slowly. Moving too quickly with a jerking action can lead to injury and means you are not getting the full benefit of the exercise.

Before you start a strengthening programme, get some advice from a cardiac rehabilitation physiotherapist.

How to Build Muscle Strength

Perform strengthening exercises at least 2 days a week. Always remember your warm-up and cool-down. Involve all the major muscle groups of the body: legs, hips, chest, abdomen, shoulders and arms (calf raises, squats, lunges, biceps curls, triceps extensions, shoulder press, chest press, pull-downs, sit-ups and lower-back extensions). There is no specific duration for strengthening exercises, but by the end you should feel muscle fatigue—as if you need a rest. For example, when lifting dumbbells or free weights, do the following:

- Include 8 to 10 different exercises in each session.
- Perform 8 to 12 repetitions with a weight that is heavy enough to make the last couple of repetitions feel difficult. By the last repetition you should feel you need to have a rest.

Flexibility

Flexibility exercise is also beneficial to your health. But remember to keep your heart healthy, add flexibility exercises to your regular aerobic exercise.

There are lots of benefits from regularly performing exercise that makes you more flexible and lots of different ways to do it. Table 5.5 outlines a few of these exercises.

TABLE 5.5   **Exercise to Improve Flexibility**

Benefits of flexibility	Types of exercise for flexibility
• Maintains joint range of movement, this helps to reduce the effects or the development of arthritis. • Allows muscles and joints to move more efficiently which reduces aches and pains. • Reduces the likelihood of muscular strains and injuries.	• Yoga • T'ai chi • Pilates • Specific stretching exercises; hold each stretch for 10-30 seconds with no bouncing; feel mild discomfort but not pain

Balance and Coordination

Balance and coordination exercises help keep you healthy and are especially important as you age.

There are many ways to improve your balance and coordination, and important reasons why we benefit from performing this type of exercise regularly. Table 5.6 lists some of the ways you can improve your balance and coordination.

TABLE 5.6   **Exercise to Improve Balance and Coordination**

Benefits of balance and coordination	Exercises for balance and coordination
• Helps to prevent you from falling (and breaking a bone or losing your confidence). • Allows you to move more freely and gives you confidence.	• T'ai chi • Yoga • Walking • Keep-fit classes • Specific balance exercise regime

If your balance is a problem for you, speak to your doctor or physiotherapist. Many programmes exist to help build balance and coordination. Some programmes are for people who have had falls or are at risk of falling.

Putting It Together

Now, make your plan. Can you see yourself doing a balanced exercise programme two or three times per week to improve aerobic fitness, strength, flexibility and balance? Following are a couple of examples to get you thinking and planning.

Example 1

> **Thoughts:** I'd love to be fit. I want to look after my heart. I'd love to lose a bit of weight round my middle and feel strong again. I remember how great I used to feel when I went swimming regularly. I used to love swimming;

things just got in the way. My friend goes to the gym and does some weights, and I'd love to do something active with my family.

Plan: I'll go to the gym once a week with my friend. I'll go swimming once a week and go for a long hill walk or cycle at the weekend with my family. This week I'll start with the gym. I'll phone my friend now and make a date. Then next week I'll add in my swim; at least I'll have set foot in the leisure centre with my friend so it won't be so daunting. And I'll talk to the family tonight about planning a walk.

Example 2

Thoughts: My job is quite stressful and I'm always short of time but I want to be fit. I want to look after my heart and get my blood pressure down. I want to tone up. I want to be a good example to my children.

Plan: I'm going to cycle to work once a week (or more if I can). I'm going to find a t'ai chi class locally; maybe there's an early morning one I can attend before work so I don't get snowed under at work and miss it. I'll start that next week. Maybe my friend from work will come; I'll set a date with her. My friend goes to a dancing class. I'm going to go with her; I'll phone her now.

What About You?

Thoughts: What exercise do you think you would enjoy? How much time do you think you'll have? What exercise did you use to enjoy in years gone by? Do you have any friends or family who exercise? Could you join them?

Plan: Write it down, talk to your family and friends and set dates. Remember: Don't do too much in one go; add one thing at a time to your routine.

Write your own list and stick it somewhere you'll see it. A blank list is available in appendix A, Planning Your Regular Exercise, for you to cut out or print out and use. Remember to get some support; involve other people. Get them to join in; they can make their own list, encourage their activity and make it fun. If you like some time just for you, do some things by yourself, too.

Creating an Active and Fit Life

Now that you understand the 3 ways to keep healthy and fit from the activity pyramid, it's time to make them happen in your everyday life. Sometimes people think they are doing enough activity and exercise to keep their bodies healthy and fit, but they are mistaken. They are usually one of three groups of people, shown in the examples that follow. Read the examples and answer honestly: Are you one of these people?

Person 1

I go to the gym on my way home from work 5 days a week . . . *but I use the lift at work and I sit all day at my desk. Come to think of it, I even have my lunch at my desk.*

This person is doing regular structured exercise but he is sitting for long periods of time, which is affecting his health. He needs to break up the periods of sitting with movement and be more active during the day (for example go for a walk at lunch time, climb the stairs, stand up and move about every hour).

Person 2a

I'm on the go all the time; I look after my grandchildren, do the housework, go up and down stairs, walk to the train and garden . . . *but I do no structured exercise. I used to love going dancing and swimming. Where did my 'me time' go?*

Person 2b

I'm very active; I'm on the go all the time at work . . . *but I do no structured exercise. I used to love cycling and hill walking. Where did my 'me time' go?*

These people have an active life but need to do some structured exercise to get even more heart benefits.

Person 3

I'm very busy—of course I'm active . . . *but I drive everywhere, read a lot, work on the computer. Come to think of it, I'm busy but I sit most of the time.*

This person is busy but she has very little physical activity at all. Being busy does not mean being active and it definitely doesn't mean being fit. Her lack of activity is affecting her health. She needs to build activity into her everyday life, accumulate 30 minutes of activity per day, and then think about what structured exercise she would enjoy.

Table 5.7 shows you some examples of people who are fulfilling all three activity and exercise messages from the activity pyramid.

The following websites offer ideas and support for your ongoing activity and exercise.

- www.walkit.com—The urban walking map and route planner that helps you get around town on foot. Get a walking route map between any two points, including your journey time
- www.activescotland.org.uk—Provides help with finding activities local to your selected postcode.
- www.bhf.org.uk/heart-health/prevention/staying-active.aspx—Provides advice on becoming active and staying active.
- www.ouractivenation.co.uk—Encourages people to take part in easy exercises, provides simple exercises to do at home and easy ways to get fit. Contains an activity finder and lots of links to other activities.

To get started, try one of the exercise programmes in appendix E. Then, create your own active life.

TABLE 5.7 **Examples of an Active Week With a Balanced, Structured Exercise Programme**

	Sit less	Active life	Balanced, structured exercise
Ahmed, age 43	Set an alarm on my computer at work to stand up and move every hour. Get up and move on every advert break when watching TV. Walk to other rooms to speak to family instead of shouting through the walls.	Use the stairs: 3 flights at work, 1 flight at home. Use the car as little as possible (try to walk or cycle short distances). Wash the car by hand. Cut the grass.	Cycle to work: 30 minutes each way (*aerobic, strengthening, balance*). Gym programme 1 time per week: cardiovascular programme, strengthening programme and stretching programme (*aerobic, strengthening, flexibility*). Yoga 1 time per week (*strengthening, flexibility, balance and coordination*). Hill walk or cycle or tennis 1 time per week with family (*aerobic, strengthening, balance*).
Mary, age 72	Put a note near my knitting to remind me to stand up every hour. Get up and move on every advert break when watching TV. Stand when I'm on the phone.	Go with my husband or my friend when they walk the dog. Do gardening. Walk to shops and get the bus back. Get off the bus 2 stops early and walk. Use the stairs. Do housework.	Walk with grandchildren 1 hour a week (*aerobic, balance*). Over-50 exercise class 2 times per week; includes weights (*aerobic, balance, flexibility, strengthening*). T'ai chi 1 time per week (*strengthening, balance, flexibility*)
Jim, age 63	Set an alarm on my phone to stand up and move every hour. Get up and move on every advert break when watching TV.	Walk dog 2 times per day. Park car 15-minute walk away from work. Use the stairs. Do DIY projects. Do housework.	Swimming 1 time per week (*aerobic, strengthening*) Golf 1 time per week (*balance, strengthening*) Gym programme 1 time per week—includes cardiovascular, strengthening and stretching programmes (*aerobic, strengthening, flexibility*). Hill walk with club 1 time per week (*aerobic, balance, strengthening*).

6

Eat Well

Food plays an important part in your life. You need it for energy, you eat it for enjoyment, it can be part of your social life and it can improve how you look and feel. So, can a healthy diet do all of these things and help to protect your heart, too? Yes! Eating well and getting the right balance of foods in your diet are important for the health of your heart and it can be enjoyable and much easier than you think.

> Since my heart attack I have made changes to my diet and can't believe how much I am enjoying my food now. I actually look forward to meal times.
>
> John, age 44

Getting the right food into your body can help to control many CHD risk factors, such as obesity, diabetes, high cholesterol and high blood pressure. The right food can therefore help to prevent or control CHD. This chapter discusses getting the right food for a healthy heart and how to do this in a practical, achievable and enjoyable way.

A Balanced Diet

What is a balanced diet? You may have seen a picture of the eatwell plate (see figure 6.1) at the hospital, doctor's surgery or during your cardiac rehabilitation programme. It shows five groups of food and how much people should eat from each group every day.

The eatwell plate applies to most people, whether they are a healthy weight or overweight, carnivore or vegetarian. It applies to people of all ethnic origins. However, it does not apply to children under 2 years of age because they have different nutritional needs. Also, if you have special dietary requirements or medical needs, you may want to check with a registered dietitian and discuss whether the eatwell plate applies to you.

The eatwell plate

Use the eatwell plate to help you get the balance right. It shows how
much of what you eat should come from each food group.

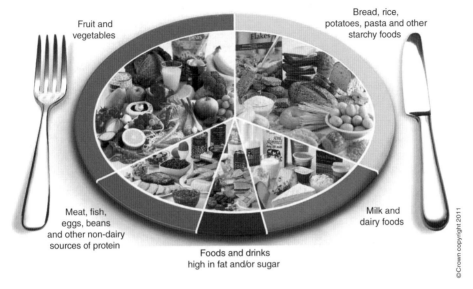

Fruit and
vegetables

Bread, rice,
potatoes, pasta and other
starchy foods

Meat, fish,
eggs, beans
and other non-dairy
sources of protein

Milk and
dairy foods

Foods and drinks
high in fat and/or sugar

©Crown copyright 2011

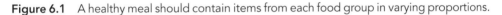

Department of Health in association with the Welsh Government, the Scottish Government and the Food Standards Agency in Northern Ireland

Figure 6.1   A healthy meal should contain items from each food group in varying proportions.

According to the eatwell plate, you need five groups of food for general health.
You need different amounts of each food group for different reasons, and the
eatwell plate shows how much of a day's food intake should come from each
group. It contains everything you eat each day, including snacks. To get a balanced diet, do the following:

1. Choose a variety of foods from each food group.
2. Keep meals and snacks interesting.
3. Avoid monotony of eating the same things every day.

Bread, Rice, Potatoes and Other Starchy Foods

These foods are nutritious and easily processed to provide your body with energy.
It is best to choose wholegrain varieties from this group (wholemeal bread, cereal,
rice or pasta) because wholegrain has more fibre and other important nutrients
such as iron and B vitamins. You can digest wholegrain foods more slowly than
refined grains, which helps to keep you fuller for longer. The fuller you feel, the
less likely you are to eat too much or reach for sugary and fatty snacks. Oats are
part of the starchy food group and have additional benefits: They contain soluble
fibre, which can help to lower LDL cholesterol. As you can see from the eatwell
plate, you should aim to have a third of your day's food intake from this group.

♥ Increase Starchy Foods in Your Diet

- Start the day with a wholegrain or oat-based cereal or mix some in with your favourite cereal.
- Have a sandwich for lunch. Choose from the many types of bread available such as poppy seed bagels and wholemeal baguettes.
- Base your main meal around potatoes, pasta, rice or grains such as couscous or bulgur wheat.
- Try to have more rice or pasta than sauce at meals.
- Maximise fibre and vitamins by leaving skins on potatoes.

Some people think this group of foods is fattening. However, gram for gram it contains fewer than half the calories of fat. Fats that people add to these foods tend to add extra calories to the diet. For example, many people add butter to bread or creamy sauces to pasta.

I always thought carbohydrate was fattening, and I tried to cut down on it. I felt peckish between meals and tended to snack. Since having a bit more carbohydrate at meals, I seem to have cut back on a few snacks because I don't feel as hungry now.

Barbara, age 58

Fruit and Vegetables

Fruit and vegetables are low in calories, are high in antioxidants and can contain soluble fibre. Most people know they need to eat more fruit and vegetables to keep healthy. When asked how many portions they should eat every day most people can answer 5 a day, but many are unsure of how big a portion is.

What Is a Portion?

A portion of fruit or vegetables is 80 grams. However, the easiest way to think of a portion is the amount you can fit in your hand: one portion equals one handful. Here are a few examples:

- 1 apple, orange, banana, pear or other similar-size fruit
- 2 smaller fruits such as plums, apricots or tangerines
- 3 heaped tablespoons of carrots, peas or sweet corn
- A handful of very small fruits such as grapes, strawberries or cherries
- A dessert bowl of salad
- A glass (150ml) of pure fruit or vegetable juice

Here are a few exceptions to the 1 portion equals 1 handful rule:

- Pure fruit juice counts as only one portion, no matter how much you have (because of skin and pulp being removed and high sugar content).
- Potatoes are not counted as vegetables; they are counted as starchy carbohydrate.
- A tablespoon of dried fruit counts as one portion.

Eating at least 5 portions of fruit and vegetables each day may be the recommended amount, but when it comes to keeping your heart healthy, the more portions the better.

♥ Finding It Difficult to Eat Five a Day?

Try to include a portion or two of fruits or vegetables at meal and snack times and it will soon add up. Try the following:

- Add a handful of berries or dried fruit or chop a banana in to cereal.
- Have a glass of pure fruit or vegetable juice with breakfast.
- Have a vegetable-based soup.
- Add salad and tomatoes into a sandwich.
- Snack on fruit or chopped vegetables.
- Have at least two handfuls of vegetables with your main meal.
- Try a fruit-based dessert using fresh, frozen or tinned varieties of fruit.

For more ideas visit www.nhs.uk/LiveWell/5ADAY.

What Are Antioxidants?

Antioxidants are vitamins and minerals found in wholegrains, fruits, and vegetables. The body produces free radicals when you perform everyday activities such as eating and breathing. Free radicals can also be caused by environment factors such as smoking, pollution and UV sunlight. Too many free radicals can cause damage to your heart and body cells. Antioxidants combine with free radicals in your body to make them harmless, thereby protecting your heart.

Whether fresh, frozen, tinned, dried or juiced, all fruit and vegetables are packed with vitamins and minerals. You can provide your heart and body with antioxidants and even more nutrients by choosing various colours and types of fruit and vegetables—and you will brighten up your meals, too!

> Antioxidants protect your heart. They are found in wholegrains, fruit and vegetables.

Milk and Dairy Foods

This food group includes milk, cheese and yoghurt. Milk and dairy foods provide protein, vitamins and calcium. Calcium is needed for many body functions such as helping the blood to clot and keeping teeth and bones strong. Try to have some foods from this group every day. However, these foods can contribute to saturated fat intake, so try to choose lower-fat varieties of these foods. Low-fat dairy foods contain just as much calcium and protein as the high-fat versions. There is a growing range of low-fat dairy foods, so it's worth trying different products. This way you can find the ones you like and the ones that are best suited to your lifestyle.

♡ Reduce Saturated Fat in Milk and Dairy Foods

- Choose semi-skimmed milk or 1 percent milk fat. They both contain all the calcium and vitamins without the added fat.
- Use low-fat natural yoghurt, Greek yoghurt or fromage frais instead of cream in recipes or with desserts and fruit.
- Use small amounts of a strong cheese such as mature cheddar or blue cheese to flavour foods. You can even grate it to make it go further.
- Alternatively, choose low-fat cheese in recipes. Low-fat cottage cheese and quark are the lowest-fat varieties of cheese.
- Try soya milk or yogurts with added calcium for a non-dairy alternative.

I have always used full-cream milk in my tea because I felt the other stuff was too watery and tasteless, but I have now gotten used to the semi-skimmed milk. It did take a while and it's the full-cream milk that doesn't taste right in my tea now.

George, age 56

Meat, Fish, Eggs, Beans and Other Non-Dairy Proteins

This group of food includes meat, meat products (such as pies, sausages and burgers), poultry, fish, eggs, pulses, soya protein and textured vegetable protein. These foods provide an excellent source of protein and iron and they are a rich source of vitamins and minerals. Try to have some food from this group every day.

Leaner cuts of meat such as chicken or turkey with the skin removed are lower in saturated fat and are therefore better choices than meat products such as sausages, burgers and pies. The latter choices tend to be higher in fat, especially saturated fat (discussed later in this chapter), and are best avoided or eaten sparingly.

Pulses such as beans, peas and lentils are great alternatives to meat because they are naturally low in fat and high in soluble fibre, protein, and vitamins and minerals.

Try to eat more fish, especially oily fish, because the omega-3 fat found in oily types of fish is another form of polyunsaturated fat (discussed later in this chapter) and are especially good for your heart. Omega-3 fats can help to keep your arteries smooth and supple, make your blood less likely to clot and can even help to keep your heart beat regular. Oily fish such as mackerel, kippers, pilchards, fresh tuna, trout, salmon and sardines are the best sources of omega-3 fatty acids in the diet. Try to eat these fish once or twice a week. If you have had a heart attack, try to make this two or three times a week.

Plant sources of omega-3 oils include rapeseed (canola) oil, linseed, flax or pumpkin seeds, soya beans, tofu and green, leafy vegetables. You can also find foods that are enriched with omega-3 fatty acids such as milk, spreads and bread. These omega-3 enriched foods usually have plant sources of omega-3 added to them. However, be aware that plant sources of omega-3 need to be converted into the type found in fish before the body can use it efficiently. The human body finds it easier to use the omega-3 found directly in fish. Try different varieties of fresh, tinned or frozen fish. You can include fish cakes and fish pies, but preferably not fish in batter because it can be high in the types of fat you should eat sparingly.

Oily Fish

- Oily fish such as mackerel, kippers, pilchards, fresh tuna, trout, salmon and sardines are the best sources of omega-3 in the diet.
- Try to eat these types of fish once or twice a week.
- If you have had a heart attack, try to make this two or three times a week. The aim is 1 g of omega-3 per day, so check labels to make sure you are getting enough.

For more information on checking labels, visit www.nhs.uk/Livewell/Goodfood/Pages/food-labelling.aspx or download the label reading leaflets from BHF and CHSS.

Eggs are a good source of protein, vitamins (especially vitamins A, D and B2) and minerals such as iodine. They can be a quick and easy meal to prepare. They contain some cholesterol; however, cholesterol-containing foods do not have a significant effect on blood cholesterol levels in most people. The saturated fats in foods have the greatest effect on blood cholesterol levels.

Eggs and Cholesterol

- Foods that contain cholesterol (such as eggs) do not have a significant effect on blood cholesterol levels.
- There are no recommendations for how many eggs you should eat. To get all the nutrients your body needs, try to eat as varied a diet as possible.
- You only need to cut down on eggs or foods high in cholesterol if you have been advised to do so by your GP or a registered dietitian.

♥ A Word About Cholesterol

- It is vital for the day-to-day functioning of the body.
- It is a fatty substance that needs to reach every cell in the body.
- It has its own transport system called lipoproteins.
- The body makes most of the cholesterol it needs in the liver.
- It mainly comes from saturated fat in the foods you eat.
- You can also get it from foods that contain cholesterol such as eggs, liver and prawns (but cholesterol in these foods does not have a significant effect on blood cholesterol levels).
- Too much LDL cholesterol causes CHD.

Foods and Drinks High in Fat or Sugar

Foods high in fat include butter, margarine, other fat spreads, oils, cream and mayonnaise. Sugar can come from sugary fizzy drinks, granulated sugar, chocolate and sweets. Some foods, such as cakes, biscuits, pastries and ice cream, are both high in fat and sugar. These foods are often high in calories and contain very few other nutrients. It is a good idea to cut down on these foods or only eat them occasionally and to get the majority of calories and nutrients your body needs from the other four food groups.

♥ Limit Fat and Sugar

This group of foods can be included as part of a balanced diet, but try the following to keep it to a minimum:

- Spread fats on to bread and crackers thinly.
- Use as little oil in cooking as possible.
- Choose lower-fat sauces, gravies and salad dressings wherever you can.
- Try to reduce or cut out sugar added to hot drinks.
- Choose diet, sugar-free or no-added-sugar drinks wherever possible.

If you do get hungry between meals try to have a healthier snack such as fruit, wholemeal toast or cereal, low-fat yoghurt or a few unsalted nuts such as almonds, macadamia nuts or pecan nuts, which all contain high levels of good monounsaturated fats.

Snacking on biscuits, crisps and chocolate late at night has always been a habit of mine; it's time to cut out the snacks and get some new habits.

Stephanie, age 62

What Does It All Mean?

At this point you understand what food groups make up a healthy, balanced diet. Now it's time to clear up any confusion about other aspects of our diet that can affect heart health. After experiencing a heart event, people commonly want to know about cholesterol, fats, salt, alcohol, food supplements and portion control.

Lowering Cholesterol

The best way to lower your cholesterol is to cut down on saturated fat and eat more foods containing soluble fibre.

Plant Stanols and Sterols

Plant stanols and sterols, also known as phytostanols and phytosterols, are naturally occurring substances found in plant foods such as fruit, vegetables, nuts and seeds. They help to lower cholesterol by blocking its absorption in the gut. They have a similar structure to cholesterol and therefore can be absorbed by the gut instead of cholesterol. They resemble the chemical structure of animal cholesterol and carry out similar functions in plants. If enough stanols or sterols are consumed in the diet, they compete with cholesterol in the digestive tract and block its absorption. Ultimately this reduces the amount of cholesterol that is absorbed in the body and returned to the liver. This can help to lower total cholesterol and the LDL cholesterol levels in the blood. Most people's diets only provide a small amount of stanols and sterols from plant foods; however, these substances are added in larger amounts to some spreads, yoghurts, yoghurt drinks and cheeses. Look out for plant stanol esters or plant sterol esters when looking at the ingredients list of these products. Research has shown that if taken on a regular basis in the recommended amounts each day, plant stanols and sterols, along with a healthy diet low in saturated fat, can help lower LDL cholesterol levels by 10 to 15 percent.

Foods With Added Plant Stanols and Sterols

- They are not substitutes for a healthy diet or cholesterol-lowering drugs.
- They must be eaten in certain amounts along with a healthy diet low in saturated fat to have an effect on cholesterol.

If you do decide to use them, follow the manufacturer's guidelines on how much of these products you need to take to achieve your 2 grams of plant stanols and sterols a day. Foods with added plant stanols and sterols are not routinely recommended because they are not suitable for everyone and their effects can vary between individuals.

For more information on plant stanols or sterols and whether they are suitable for you, contact a registered dietitian or visit www.bda.uk.com/foodfacts.

Facts About Fat

Small amounts of fat are essential to a healthy diet; you need fat in your diet to help absorb vitamins A, D, E and K in your body. Fat contains more calories per gram (9 kcal/g) than carbohydrate (3.75 kcal/g) or protein (4 kcal/g). This means that foods containing high amounts of fat tend to be high in calories, so eating large amounts can lead to weight gain and obesity. Most people consume too much fat.

In order to keep your heart healthy you should watch the amount of fat and the types of fats you eat. Fats are made up of a substance called fatty acids. The three main types of fatty acids are saturated, monounsaturated and polyunsaturated. The foods you eat contain a mixture of these fatty acids; however, the food is often grouped by the fatty acid that is most prominent within the food. For example, butter is called a saturated fat because it contains mostly saturated fatty acids, olive oil is called monounsaturated fat because it contains mostly monounsaturated fatty acids and vegetable oils are called polyunsaturated fats because they mainly contain polyunsaturated fatty acids.

> In order to keep your heart healthy you should watch the amount of fat and the types of fat you eat.

Saturated Fat

Cutting down on saturated fat can help you lower your blood cholesterol and lower your risk of heart disease. This type of fat is often solid at room temperature. Main sources are butter, fatty meat, meat products, full-fat dairy foods, cakes, biscuits, pastries and savoury snacks.

Monounsaturated Fat

Try to replace saturated fats with this type of fat to help lower LDL cholesterol without affecting our HDL cholesterol. Main sources are olive oil, rapeseed oil, avocados, nuts and seeds.

Polyunsaturated Fat

This type of fat helps to lower cholesterol levels and can be enjoyed in small amounts. Main sources are from sunflower, vegetable oils and spreading fats made from these oils. Oil-rich fish such as salmon, trout, mackerel, pilchards and sardines are also good sources of these fats.

Trans Fat

Trans fat is another type of fatty acid naturally found in small amounts in meat and dairy products. It can also be made and added to foods such as manufactured biscuits, cakes, and pastries and are found in fried foods in restaurants and takeaways. In this form it can act like saturated fat and raise your LDL cholesterol. Avoid trans fat in this form as much as possible. In recent years the food industry has reduced the amount of trans fat used in food products, but always read labels on packaged food to know what you are eating.

 How to Cut Down on Saturated Fat

The type of meat product you choose and how you cook it can make a big difference to the saturated fat content. To cut down on saturated fat, try the following:

- Limit processed meats such as sausages, burgers and pies because they can often be high in fat and salt.
- Choose leaner cuts of meat and mince.
- Cut the fat off meat and skin off poultry before cooking.
- Grill, bake or poach meat, poultry and fish. Don't fry.
- Boil, poach or scramble an egg.
- Try to have a meat-free day and choose pulses, beans, eggs or soya protein instead.

For more information on soya and health visit www.bda.uk.com/foodfacts/soya_and_health.pdf.

Cutting Down on Salt

High intakes of salt have been linked with high blood pressure. Sodium is the main ingredient in salt. Other sources of sodium include stock cubes, soy sauce, cured meats and cheese. Snack foods such as crisps, salted nuts and pickled foods can also contain high levels of sodium in the form of salt. Cut down on processed food or ready-made meals; they are often high in salt. Preparing and cooking your own meals will naturally cut down on salt.

Alternatives With Lower or Reduced Salt

- These products still taste salty and contain sodium.
- Some people find they don't taste the same and add more salt to compensate!
- It is better gradually use less salt and let your taste buds adjust. Or, flavour your foods with pepper, herbs, spices or lemon juice instead.

Reduced-salt alternatives are not suitable for some people, such as those with heart failure or kidney problems. Consult your doctor or health professional before using these products.

Why not try some of the recipes provided in appendix C? Choose foods lower in salt and avoid adding extra salt to cooking or at the table. Rediscover the real taste of your favourite foods. Try adding flavour with herbs, spices, lemon juice or black pepper. Adults should aim for no more than 6 grams, or 1 level teaspoon, of salt each day.

For more information on how to cut down on salt visit www.eatwell.gov.uk/salt.

Alcohol

Moderate amounts of alcohol have been shown to offer some protection for men over 40 years of age and post-menopausal women who have CHD. This evidence is based on people drinking just one or two units of alcohol a day. However, this does not mean that nondrinkers should start taking alcohol. There are healthier ways to protect your heart, such as adopting a healthy diet, increasing your physical activity and stopping smoking, as discussed in chapter 3.

Calculating Units of Alcohol

To work out how many units are in any drink, multiply the total volume of drink (in ml) by its strength ABV (alcohol by volume; this is measured as a percentage) and divide the result by 1,000:

Strength (ABV) × volume (ml) ÷ 1,000 = units of alcohol

For example, to work out the number of units in a pint (568 ml) of strong lager (ABV 5.2%):

5.2% × 568 ml ÷ 1,000 = 2.95 units of alcohol

Aim to keep to within recommended daily amounts of alcohol:

3-4 units alcohol for men.

2-3 units alcohol for women.

Try to have at least a couple of alcohol-free days in the week.

Alcohol is also high in calories, so cutting down could help to control your weight.

Excessive alcohol consumption can increase blood pressure, triglycerides and can have an impact on weight and body shape. Alcohol is not recommended for some heart conditions and with certain medications. Check with your doctor or pharmacist if it is safe for you to drink alcohol.

For the facts and more information on units and alcohol visit www.drinkaware.co.uk.

Getting the Right Amount of Food

Everyone needs different amounts of energy in the form of calories (kcal) from food in order to maintain a healthy weight and shape. How much you need can depend on many factors including your height, your weight and how active you are. On average women of normal, healthy weight need about 2,000kcal each day and men need about 2,500kcal each day. If you consume more calories than your body uses, then you put on weight. The reason is that the body stores any unused energy, usually as fat. It only takes a small amount of extra energy each day to put on weight over time. It can lead to becoming overweight or obese. The good news is the converse is true, too: Cutting out a little bit each day can lead to weight loss over time. For easy food swaps to help you cut extra calories and fat from your diet, see appendix B at the end of the book. Small changes can make a big difference over time.

A Word About Supplements

Most people can get all the nutrients they need from a healthy diet. The body is designed to absorb food and supplements can't do the same job as a balanced diet. However, some people may need certain supplements. For example, people aged over 65 or are of Asian origin or rarely go outdoors should consider taking a vitamin D supplement and strict vegans may consider taking a vitamin B12 supplement. For more information talk to your GP or another health professional or visit www.nhs.uk/news/2011/05May/Documents/BtH_supplements.pdf.

Since I've quit smoking, everything tastes so much better; the problem now is eating too much good food.

Peter, age 48

Refer to figure 3.3 to check whether you are at a healthy weight. If you are worried about your weight, ask your GP or dietitian for advice on how to safely lose weight and to maintain a healthy weight. For more information on how to lose weight the healthy way, visit www.nhs.uk/Livewell/Loseweight.

Is Your Relationship Bad for You?

When it comes to food portions, size really does matter. As a general rule, men tend to need more calories a day than women. If we eat the same portion as our partner we may be eating too much.

Keep Going for Life

Everyone has different reasons for deciding to eat healthy. Protecting your heart after a CHD diagnosis is one very good reason for adopting a healthy eating pattern for life. Following the eatwell plate will help you on your way to a healthy heart. The eatwell plate is all about the foods you can eat rather than what you can't eat. It will become easier over time to follow the eatwell plate; it can even become a habit. Having regular meals and foods from the four main food groups in the eatwell plate will help to keep you feeling full and less likely to reach for those sugary and fatty snacks. Keep in mind that your diet should be balanced, not boring. Appendix C offers some interesting and healthy recipes for you to try.

Don't worry if you have a lapse and eat more or you eat something you wish you hadn't; it's normal to do that sometimes. There are no forbidden foods in the eatwell plate. It gives you the flexibility to choose food you and your family often already eat and enjoy. And foods such as crisps, cakes and chocolate can be included now and then. Even the odd glass of wine or beer is allowed if you fancy it. Once you have made up your mind to make changes to your diet, set goals to help you make those changes (see table 6.1). You are more likely to achieve goals if you are involved in creating them and you set them for yourself.

For more individual advice on you and your diet, ask your doctor, practice nurse or cardiac rehabilitation team to refer you to a dietitian. For more information on healthy eating, visit www.nhs.uk/livewell/healthy-eating.

TABLE 6.1   SMART Goals Are the Smart Way to Go

Specific	Decide what you want to achieve and how you will achieve it. Instead of just setting the goal *I am going to start eating healthy,* think about what specifically you are going to do to eat healthy. Specific goals related to eating healthy include *I will start eating breakfast every day; at lunch I will swap crisps with fruit* or *I will cut the fat off meat before cooking.*
Measurable	Put a number to it. By putting a number to it you will be able to check if you are on target to achieving your goal. Measurable goals related to eating healthy include *I will eat at least two portions of fruit every day* and *I will eat a portion of fish every week.*
Achievable	Start small so your goal is achievable. The more realistic the goal, the easier it is to achieve. Making small, gradual changes makes it easier to accept and easier to reach your final goal. Examples of achievable goals related to eating healthy include *I will have an extra portion of vegetables with my evening meal* and *I will serve meals on smaller plates.*
Relevant	Make sure your goal makes sense and is relevant to you. If you do not add salt to cooking or on meals at the table, cutting down on salt does not make sense. Examples of relevant goals related to eating healthy include *I drink too many sugary drinks so I will cut sugar out of my tea* and *I will swap sugary cola for diet cola.*
Timed	Give yourself a deadline, such as every day, every morning or twice a week. Deadlines make it easier for you to manage if you have achieved your goals. Instead setting the goal *I am going to lose half a stone in weight,* try *I will lose a pound a week and in 7 weeks I will have lost half a stone* or *I will have 3 planned meals a day.*

Food plays a big part in people's lives. It provides energy and nutrients to the body and it is also part of social life. Food is such a big part of life, from providing the body with energy and nutrients to being a part of our social lives. So remember to enjoy it!

Cope With Stress and Learn to Relax

Being told you have had a heart attack or that you have a heart condition is stressful. Going through major heart surgery puts a lot of stress on your body and mind. In addition, modern life is stressful. We're often doing 10 things at once, juggling many jobs and responsibilities. You can't take stress out of life and you probably wouldn't want to. A reasonable amount of stress is actually good for you; it keeps you alert and interested in life and it helps you to achieve things. But if stress becomes overwhelming and you feel out of control, then it can have negative effects on your physical and emotional health.

> Learning to relax and cope with stress aids in recovery after a heart event and in maintaining good health in the future.

Think About a Guitar

- If the strings are too loose, they won't play good music.
- If the strings are too tight, they won't play good music and might even break.
- If the strings are tuned just right, they will play good music as long as they are kept in tune.
- You need to have just enough stress in your life to keep alert and able to achieve things, but not so much that you snap. Therefore, you must take steps to keep balanced.

If you have had a heart event and you are trying to cope with lots of other stresses at the same time (such as money, relationships, job), it's even more important that you try to do as much as you can to help your body and mind cope and that you don't let stress become distressful. This is easier said than done.

It's not as simple to de-stress as you might think; sometimes it's just life. But you have to do your best and keep practising your relaxation, just like any change in your lifestyle. Keep trying; it doesn't happen overnight, but it does help.

Ian, age 76

You can try to keep on top of stress by learning to pay attention to your body. Often it tells you when stress is building up or when you are not coping well. But before discussing how to cope or how to relax, you must understand what stress is and how it affects you.

Defining Stress

Stress is a normal part of life. People feel stressed by little things such as traffic jams and shopping queues, and people feel stressed by big things such as health, money, work, family, relationships and moving house. When stressed by something or someone, the body releases hormones (adrenaline and cortisol) that make you prepare to stay and fight or run away from the stress; this is called the fight-or-flight response. This response is the body's automatic reaction, or a natural stress response. These hormones make you ready for action; they prepare you to fight or flee in the following ways:

- They release fats and sugars into your blood to give you more energy.
- They make your muscles tense up.
- They make you sweat more and your mouth dry.
- They make your heart beat faster and your blood pressure rise in order to carry more blood to your muscles and brain.
- They make you breathe faster, increasing the amount of oxygen in your body.
- They heighten senses, making them more alert.

How Stress and Distress Affect the Health of Your Heart

It's easy and actually unhelpful to blame stress for your heart event. People commonly want to blame stress but it's important that you do not ignore other areas of your lifestyle.

I know I smoke, which didn't help, but the main thing that caused my heart attack was stress.

Louise, age 54

Hard work by itself doesn't cause stress or heart attacks. But if you don't allow yourself to take time for enjoyment or relaxation you put your body and mind under more stress than it was designed to cope with. It's also possible to work hard and remain relaxed. You can learn to pay attention to tension and control your response to stress.

One can't say for sure that stress can cause heart disease. The trouble starts when you feel out of control or you feel under stress all the time without time to relax. Adrenaline levels are constantly high, causing tension and anxiety. If you regularly feel overwhelmed and worn down by stress, in other words if you feel distressed a lot of the time, then you are more likely to reach for things that you think will help you to cope or give you comfort such as high-fat foods, alcohol or cigarettes. This increases your CHD risk factors. Table 7.1 details the physical effects stress has on the inside of the body and also how it influences our behaviour on the outside.

TABLE 7.1   When Stress Becomes Prolonged, Overwhelming and Distressing

What's happening on the outside	What's happening on the inside
• You eat more high-fat and comforting foods. • You 'don't have time' for activity and exercise. • You put on weight. • You smoke more cigarettes. • You drink too much alcohol.	• High heart rate and blood pressure • High cholesterol and blood sugar levels • Increase in blood clotting • Increased inflammation in the artery walls • Higher risk of constriction of coronary arteries • Higher risk of an irregular heart rhythm

Too much stress makes it harder to change unhealthy behaviours such as smoking, eating an unhealthy diet, inactivity or drinking too much alcohol. It's common for people to think that smoking, drinking too much alcohol, being inactive and 'comfort' eating makes them feel less stressed; however, the relief is only temporary. In the long term, these behaviours will have a negative impact on your general health and the health of your heart. So, it's important to learn to cope with stress more effectively, reduce the effects of stress and help yourself to choose a healthy future.

How You Can Help Yourself

Learning ways to cope with stress prevents it from becoming distressful and harmful to you. To help yourself cope in a healthy way, do the following:

- Keep an eye on your stress levels. Ask yourself what makes you stressed.
- Listen to your body.
- Do more of the things that help you to relax and that make you feel happy and positive.

The following sections explain these coping strategies in more detail.

Knowing What Makes You Stressed

The most common causes of stress are health problems and worries, work, money problems, relationships, family, marriage, divorce, unemployment, moving house, bereavement, time pressure and loneliness. Often people deal with many of these things all at once. Often people have difficulty accepting that they are struggling to cope with stress. Sometimes people are unaware of stress, often as a result of hectic daily routines that are steadily draining.

You cannot always control the stressors in your life, but you can control how you respond to them. The way you think about things has a powerful effect on how you cope with stress. If you assume the worst all the time without knowing the facts, you can cause your own distress. For example, after a heart attack or being told they have angina, some people make their own minds up about what this is and what it means for their future. People are often misguided by advice from well-meaning friends and neighbours or they may have misunderstood something that was said to them by a health professional. Constantly having negative thoughts and assuming the worst for the future generates more stress, therefore it's important to ask questions. Don't be misguided by your own thoughts; clarify information with a health professional.

It's normal for stress levels to go up and down much like the temperature over a period of time. One way to keep an eye on your stress levels is to picture a stress thermometer (see figure 7.1); instead of measuring temperature, it measures how you are feeling, your stress levels or your adrenaline levels. The words in the stress thermometer describe how your feelings change as your adrenaline levels go up and down.

It's normal for stress levels to be higher after a heart event. People often feel tense or have a bad temper for a while. If you constantly feel tense, bad-tempered, worried, scared or in a panic without time to relax, then it may well be having a negative effect on your health. Health problems start when stress levels are high all day, and day after day. Think about why you are feeling this way. Are you worried about your health? Are you worrying about specific symptoms related to your health? Are you worried about a relationship? Are you worried about your

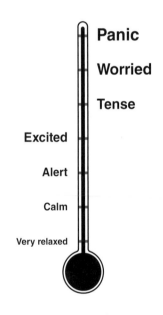

Figure 7.1 The stress thermometer shows how we feel as adrenaline goes up. As it does we move from deeply relaxed—to wide awake—to excited. If it goes up too much more it makes us feel tense, bad tempered, tired, pressurised, fed up and so on.

work or money? Are you worried about lots of things? This can help you to identify which are the areas of greatest concern, providing a good starting point for developing a plan to address the concerns. This chapter includes many ideas to help your body to cope and encourage these feelings to pass. These relaxation techniques are then discussed in more detail later in this chapter. Use the list in appendix A, Coping with Stress, to help you pinpoint and write down your stressors and how you plan to manage them.

Listening to Your Body

Your body will 'tell' you if you are starting to struggle with too much stress. Table 7.2 outlines common responses to stress. Do more things that help you to relax, de-stress and feel happy and positive.

TABLE 7.2 **How Your Body Responds to Too Much Stress**

Physical reactions and symptoms	Behaviour
<ul><li>Shallow breathing</li><li>Tense muscles; aching neck and back</li><li>Clenching your jaw; grinding your teeth</li><li>Inability to sit for long, stand queues or wait</li><li>Sweating or trembling</li><li>Headache</li><li>Ringing in the ears</li><li>Heart beating faster, chest pain</li><li>Butterflies in your stomach, tight or knotty feelings in your stomach, needing to go to the toilet more</li><li>Loss of appetite for food, fun or sex</li></ul>	<ul><li>Poor lifestyle: overeating, smoking, too much alcohol, feeling too tired to exercise</li><li>Always rushing</li><li>Neglecting personal appearance</li><li>Withdrawing from relationships or social situations</li><li>Starting tasks and not finishing them; restlessness</li><li>Oversleeping or not sleeping, disturbed nights, waking early, nightmares</li><li>Poor performance at work</li><li>Taking lots of sick leave</li></ul>
Emotions	Your brain and your thoughts
<ul><li>Impatient, snapping at people, irritable, short-tempered, tendency to criticise and argue, moodiness</li><li>Lack of sense of humour</li><li>Tearful, unhappy, sad, sense of paranoia, more sensitive than normal</li><li>Feeling lonely</li><li>Feeling overwhelmed</li><li>Feeling that there just aren't enough hours in the day</li><li>Loss of self-esteem; feelings of worthlessness</li></ul>	<ul><li>Constantly frustrated or annoyed</li><li>Forgetful, poor memory</li><li>Lack of interest</li><li>Poor concentration</li><li>Seeing only the negative; worrying</li><li>Racing thoughts, anxious</li><li>'I can't do this'.</li><li>'I can't cope'.</li><li>'Everything is pointless'.</li></ul>

Practicing Relaxation and Positive Thinking

Relaxation is letting go of tension in the body and mind. It can help you feel peaceful and calm. Practicing a relaxation technique regularly has been shown to reduce anxiety, which can make a big difference in your life. Doing something regularly that you find relaxing has many positive benefits to your general health and the health of your heart.

Benefits of Regular Relaxation

- It lowers blood pressure and heart rate.
- It can help to control the discomfort of angina and breathlessness.
- It helps you to feel more confident in making changes in your behaviour, such as stopping smoking, eating healthily, exercising regularly and not drinking too much alcohol.
- It can help you to sleep better.
- It can help you to have more energy.
- It helps you to get through a busy day less stressed and tired.
- It helps you to cope better with everyday problems such as work, difficult relationships and pain.
- It helps you to cope better with irritability and frustration.
- It helps you deal with the urge to rush all the time.
- It helps you reduce muscle aches and tiredness.
- It makes you more effective at the things you have to do.

There are lots of ideas of how you can help yourself manage stress in table 7.3. Some of the suggestions might seem too simple or even offbeat, but they all work! The key to your success is to find something that you enjoy and that works for you. Then, make time to do it regularly. But if you feel that you are doing all you can to help yourself and you are still feeling regularly overwhelmed and worn down, then you must speak to a health professional. The rest of this chapter teaches you how to tackle stress with relaxation techniques, some of which are summarized in table 7.3.

I didn't realise how tense I was. Practising my relaxation CD has made me aware of where I hold tension.

Margaret, age 71

I make sure I go for a walk every lunchtime. I didn't realize how important me time could be.

Moira, age 59

TABLE 7.3 Ways to Cope With Stress in Everyday Life

Stress-reducing lifestyle choices	Stress-reducing relaxation techniques
• Eat well • Keep physically active (e.g., regular walks, t'ai chi, yoga, Pilates). • Keep alcohol to within healthy limits (see chapter 6). • Don't smoke. • Slow down; make time for rest and relaxation. • Get enough sleep. • Manage your time; learn to say no. • Make time for yourself. • Talk; ask for help. • Avoid too many stimulants. • Switch off the TV. • Get a pet.	• Breathe deeply. • Listen to your body; pay attention to tension. Try positive talk; think of your own mantra. • Use a relaxation CD regularly. • Use progressive muscular relaxation— PMR. • Use meditation. Use mindfulness. • Spend relaxing time with friends and family. Talk and laugh! • Take a warm bath. • Enjoy a relaxing hobby. • Listen to music, enjoy a good book or read the paper. • Go for a massage.

Breathe Deeply

You may not be able to control the things that add stress to your life but you can control your breathing. Deep breathing promotes a relaxation response and is an effective calming technique during a stressful situation. You can also practise it throughout the day to help prevent tension and stress. Deep breathing is also known as diaphragmatic breathing (breathing using your diaphragm). If you're just learning deep breathing you should practice it lying down first. Then when it becomes natural to you, you'll be able to do it anywhere, anytime.

Deep Breathing

- Start by closing your eyes. Uncurl your fingers and toes and wiggle them to relieve tension. Open your teeth slightly to relax your jaw. Let your tummy muscles relax (let them go).
- Take a few normal breaths.
- Now, each time you breathe try to breathe out a little bit further; this will automatically make you take a deeper breath in.
- Don't force it. It should be a comfortable, slow, long breath in. Hold it for a second. Then take a comfortable, slow, longer breath out (think about doing a long sigh as you exhale).
- Feel your tummy expanding as you breathe in and getting smaller as you breathe out; feel your belly rise and fall with your breath.
- Eventually your breathing will naturally fall into an even, long, slow rhythm.
- Feel your shoulders relax and feel the tension leave your body each time you breathe out slowly.

Pay Attention to Tension

You can learn to spot tension if you start checking for it. This is called rapid relaxation or a body scan. Some people find it helpful to use something to remind them to check for tension and help them get into the habit of checking for tension. For example, you can put a dot on your watch, a sticker on your computer or an alarm on your phone. Try to practise this 15 to 20 times per day and it will become natural for you to notice tension and let it go. Once you are very familiar with what tension feels like, you can even control tension while you are engaging in an activity or going about your everyday life. Learn to move without tension, as in t'ai chi.

Body Scan: Finding the Tension and Letting It Go

- Are my toes curled up in my shoes? Uncurl them.
- Are my knees stiff and straight? Soften them.
- Are my fingers clenched tight in fists? Unclench them.
- Are my arms stiff and straight? Soften the elbows.
- Are my shoulders tense and raised? Lower them.
- Are my teeth clenched? Open your teeth slightly and relax your jaw.
- Is my face and forehead tense and stiff? Soften your forehead and soften the muscles around your eyes.

Positive Talk

Positive talk can be a powerful stress-reducing technique. Make an effort to be aware of your own negative thoughts. When you assume the worst all the time, you can cause your own distress. To combat this tendency, create a mantra for yourself that has personal meaning and makes you feel empowered. A mantra is a phrase or sound that you repeat to yourself. For example, as you breathe in and out during relaxation and throughout your day, repeat to yourself an empowering phrase such as *I am relaxed, I am strong, I am happy, I am healthy, I am calm* or *I am in control.*

- Turn your negative thoughts into positive talk.
- Switch off the adrenaline.
- Reduce tension, worry, anxiety, stress and fear.
- Think of your own mantra: I am relaxed, I am strong, I am happy, I am healthy, I am calm or I am in control.

Avoid Stimulants

Stimulants such as caffeine make tension worse. More than 4 cups of coffee or tea a day is too much. Look out for caffeine in soft drinks, too; try the decaffeinated versions instead. Try to avoid caffeine after 6 p.m. to help you to relax properly in the evening and sleep more deeply.

Also try to avoid too much alcohol. Alcohol in moderation (2-3 units for a woman and 3-4 for a man) can feel relaxing; however, drinking too much makes it difficult to relax, sleep deeply and feel positive. Equally, overstimulation with television and computers makes it difficult to focus on the present, relax and sleep deeply.

Be Active

Being active releases happy hormones called endorphins, which reduce anxiety and frustration. Activity makes you breathe more deeply and eases muscle tension, which helps you to relax. Go for a walk, do t'ai chi, practise yoga, do Pilates or perform stretching exercises.

Learn to Say No

Practise saying no at work, to family and to friends. This is difficult for some people. You may feel guilty, but doing it can help you get control of your workload. Learn to manage your time better. Always expect things to take longer than they do. Allow more time than you need so that if things go wrong you're not stressed. Write lists; doing so is immediately calming.

Slow down

Do you work fast, struggle to sit still, get annoyed in queues, finish meals quickly, finish people's sentences? Some people seem to be born speedy but sometimes it can become a habit; people become addicted to adrenaline. To help slow down, tell yourself to take things more slowly. Use deep breathing throughout your day. Notice tension and then let it go. Practise moving more slowly and practise eating more slowly. Take pleasure in your work; take time to relax and enjoy it. Add 10 minutes on to journeys. Notice your surroundings.

Use a Relaxation CD

Using a relaxation CD is a good way to learn how to relax more deeply. You can find some relaxation techniques on the websites in appendix F or you can order a CD from the British Heart Foundation. There are many different types of relaxation. Try a few of them and get to know which one works for you. Keep in mind that relaxation is a skill and takes time to learn, so don't expect too much too soon and don't give up on one technique too soon. Plenty of practice will help you get a lasting benefit. The more you practise, the easier it becomes. Then you can use relaxation to deal with tension anytime and anywhere.

Progressive Muscular Relaxation

Tension can become so habitual that you don't notice it anymore. Progressive muscular relaxation (PMR) makes you more aware of tension in your muscles, so you can spot early warning signs of stress before it builds up. PMR is the most widely researched type of relaxation technique in people who have had a heart event. In order to become familiar and effective in using PMR you should try to practise it twice daily. Once you become familiar with the principles of PMR you can use it in your everyday life. Find PMR resources within the websites in appendix F.

Practice Mindfulness

Mindfulness is the practice of being present, calm and non-judgemental in a frantic world. Mindfulness-based stress reduction (MBSR) and mindfulness-based cognitive therapy (MBCT) are proven techniques in learning to cope with stress, anxiety and depression. This practice teaches you to understand stress, breath healthily and notice your thoughts, feelings and bodily sensations. This helps you to react to stress in a more healthy way. The practice involves meditation and can be introduced into everyday life. Find mindfulness resources within the websites in appendix F.

How to Ask for Help From Others

Whatever is worrying you, try not to hold it inside. Talk about your thoughts and feelings or write them down in a diary. Sometimes people think that talking about problems is negative when in fact it is a positive step to making things better. Even if it's hard at the time it will make things better in the long term. Talk to a friend or colleague at work. Maybe you can help each other. If you have concerns about your health speak with your doctor, practice nurse or cardiac rehabilitation professional. If you are unwell and can't go to work, speak with your doctor, practice nurse or cardiac rehabilitation professional; they might know of local agencies that can help. Ask for help and advice if you have money worries; contact the Government's National Debtline at 0808 808 4000. The Citizens' Advice Bureau can give you advice on financial or housing problems; look them up in your local phone book.

If you would like to learn more about coping with stress, a range of websites that provide self-help information on stress, including relaxation techniques, is available in appendix F. Some of these websites allow you to download audio or visual files demonstrating relaxation techniques on to your computer or other electronic device. Some also allow you to print off instructions on relaxation techniques. Many relaxation techniques are available. Breathing techniques, PMR and mindfulness are good places to start, but experiment to see what suits you.

Get Going
and Keep Going

Only 50 percent of people who join a gym stick with it and are still attending regularly after 6 months. You could be one of this 50 percent, but it will require some effort, self-discipline and a bit of time.

The modern world is an instant world—instant food, instant money, instant communication. People have learned to expect things instantly. Many of the effects of regular exercise, healthy eating, stopping smoking and coping well with stress don't happen instantly. People give up too quickly. Many of the benefits of living a healthy lifestyle cannot be seen at all; there is no visual feedback, but it is happening. You therefore need to remind yourself *why* you exercise regularly, *why* you choose the healthy food, *why* you take time to go for a walk or go to t'ai chi, *why* you don't pick up the cigarette. Make sure you and your family are in the 50 percent who stay with it and live a healthy, happy, long life!

> It wasn't easy; many of the things they asked me to change I really enjoyed. I really liked my pipe. But once I decided I needed to stop smoking, it got easier. I got some help from the smoking-cessation nurse at my health centre. I haven't smoked for 8 months now! I saved the money and I took my wife and grandchildren to a fun park. It was a great day out!
>
> William, age 65

Changing a habit is hard; staying changed is even harder. Even though it's hard, you can do it!

Staying Motivated

Now that you have more knowledge and a better understanding of the importance of adopting a healthy lifestyle, the next step is to make positive changes that will last forever. It's time for you to decide

- what you want to change,
- why it is important to you,
- what's stopping you,
- how to make a realistic plan,
- where to get support, and
- how to expect slip-ups but still feel good about your achievements.

Let's look in more detail at how to make lasting changes to your lifestyle.

What You Want to Change and Why

You are more likely to be successful in changing a behaviour if you have your own reasons. People do things when they believe it is beneficial to them and those closest to them. What's important to you? The following are examples from other people's goals. You may have similar ones, but make your own mind up.

- I want to be fitter and be able to play with my grandchildren.
- I want to stop smoking for good and help my friend to do the same.
- I want to eat more healthily and encourage my family as well.
- I want to feel less stressed all the time and be able to enjoy time with my partner.

How Important Is Change to You

A good way to motivate yourself to change a behaviour is to weigh up the positives and negatives. This lets you see how important it is. Look at table 8.1 to see how Wendy weighs the pros and cons of becoming more active.

What's Stopping You

By weighing up the positives and negatives you'll probably find out what's stopping you. Is it money? Is it time? Is it the weather? Is it a sore knee like Wendy? There's always a solution; look at the example in table 8.2.

Try it yourself. Pick a behaviour that you have thought of changing or are trying to change. Fill out the pros and cons. What's more important? What's stopping you? Get some support; talk it over with a friend or family member. Do you need some advice from a health professional?

TABLE 8.1   **Wendy (55) Wants to Feel Fitter and Is Thinking of Going Cycling Regularly**

Pros	Cons
• It's good for my heart and will help to stop me having a heart attack again.	• I'm lazy.
• It'll help me tone up.	• I don't have much time.
• I'll feel fitter and stronger.	• I'm worried about exercising with my sore knee.
• I'll have better general health.	
• I'll have more energy.	
• I'll feel happier and less stressed.	
• My children will stop nagging!	
• I can do it with my family and have more quality time with them.	

Find a blank copy of this form to copy, cut out and use in appendix A.

Make a Realistic Plan

Ask yourself the question *How confident am I about becoming more active?* To increase your confidence it's important that you set yourself some realistic goals or plans. Make sure you are specific with what you plan to do and make sure your plans are achievable. Don't just think about it; set yourself a specific time. When you are successful and achieve your goals, no matter how small they are you will feel much more confident and motivated to keep it going.

Where to Get Support

Another positive step is to get support from people you value. Involve your friends and family in your plans. You can motivate them to adopt a healthy lifestyle and you can support each other. And remember to recognise your achievements; reward yourself for your hard work. For example, if you quit smoking use the money you saved on cigarettes and go on a holiday with your family. If you have gone for regular walks with your friend for a month, notice how good you feel and plan other social events together.

Expect Slip-Ups

Don't beat yourself up. If your healthy behaviour slips, don't panic; a lapse does not mean you have failed. Everyone struggles to maintain the healthy behaviour. Missing a session at the gym or smoking a cigarette or eating something you wish you hadn't are not complete failures. Don't panic and don't beat yourself up; this is normal. Sometimes things happen that are out of your control or that take you out of your routine or weaken your determination. For example, bad weather, illness, family commitments, a holiday, a stressful time, or work commitments can challenge your goals. Don't give up. Remember all the reasons why you made the change in the first place. Don't let one lapse become a week or a month of lapses. Get back to your healthy routine the next day.

Tables 8.3a and 8.3b show you a couple of real-life situations where people are changing their lifestyle.

TABLE 8.2   Goal: 'I Want to Be Active and Fit'

Ask yourself the following questions (even better, write down your answers)

Why do I want to be fit?

I want to be fit so I have more energy in my everyday life.

I want to be active and fit to help keep my blood pressure down and help keep my heart healthy.

What activity have I enjoyed in the past?

I used to love walking, cycling and dancing.

What activity and exercise can I see myself doing now? When will I do it? Who will I do it with? (Phone them. Make it definite—a specific day and time. Don't try to do too much too soon; add one new thing at a time.)

My friend goes dancing. I'm going to phone her now and make a plan to go with her. And I'll see if any of the girls at work want to go for a walk at lunchtime. Great, I'm organised. I'm going dancing with Mary on Wednesday nights starting next week. And June and I are going to walk for half an hour at lunchtime on Mondays and Fridays starting tomorrow.

What things might stop me—weather, money, busy at work, busy with family?

I'm going to ask everyone to club together on my birthday to get me an exercise bike, then no matter what I've got a way of being active.

I'm going to do different activities with the seasons—hill walk in the summer and gym in the winter.

I'm going to go to the gym with my friend but if money gets tight we will go out for a walk or a jog at the same time as we would be at the gym so we don't break the routine.

I'm going to walk or cycle to work, which won't add much time onto my day.

I'm going to get the kids bikes so we can do that together.

What will I do when I'm out of my usual routine?

I'm going to make sure we go for walks or hire bikes on holiday so that I can keep active and feel good.

How will you reward yourself for your efforts?

I'm going to plan a special night out with my wife once I've been going to the gym regularly for 4 weeks.

Find a blank copy of this form to copy, cut out and use in appendix A.

TABLE 8.3a Becoming Active—a Real Life Situation (Frances, 46)

Week 1	I have decided to go to the gym; my target is twice per week.
Week 2	Going well; really enjoying it! My friend Sally is coming too.
Week 4	Spoke to Sally and made a plan to go tomorrow.
Week 6	Going well again; enjoying the gym. Went swimming with my husband.
Week 7	Spoke to Sally on phone; we feel really motivated. Now my husband wants to go for a cycle at the weekend with the kids.
Week 11	Still at the gym twice per week and swimming once per week with my husband. Trying to do something active with the kids at the weekend. I feel really confident!
Week 14	Loving the exercise; we all feel great! Going on holiday in a couple of months and planning to hire bikes.

→→→ Week 3
←←← Got really busy at work and missed the gym this week.

TABLE 8.3b Stopping Smoking—a Real Life Situation (Mat, 52)

Week 1	I've decided to stop smoking again! I've been to the smoking-cessation class at my health centre. I'm using patches.
Week 2	Going well; I've not smoked! I'm just trying to distract myself when I feel like having a cigarette. I'm going for lots of walks and eating lots of mints!
Week 4	Spoke to my smoking-cessation counselor (Cathy). She was great. She told me not to beat myself up and I've just got to keep reminding myself all the reasons why I want to stop. She advised me to bargain with myself if I feel like a cigarette: I can tell myself I can have it in 10 minutes once I've phoned my friend and before I know it an hour has gone by. I didn't need the cigarette. I'm determined not to smoke tomorrow.
Week 6	Going well again. I have decided to go to another class.
Week 7	Spoke with Cathy. It really helps to have support. Davie is thinking of giving up too.
Week 11	Still not smoking, I feel much better and more confident this time!
Week 14	No smoking, and I hardly miss it. Went to pub with Davie; did not smoke! He's starting his smoking-cessation class in 4 weeks.

→→→ Week 3
←←← Went to pub with Davie for a drink and had a cigarette; I feel really bad!

The website www.livinglifetothefull.com has free modular courses devised to help people develop key life skills to tackle common problems. The materials use modern educational techniques and the evidence-based cognitive behaviour therapy (CBT) approach to help bring about helpful change.

Top Tips for Keeping Active

The following useful advice will help you make activity and exercise part of your life forever.

Have Fun! Some people really like to exercise with others while some people prefer to be on their own; some people like a mixture depending on their mood. Some people love to be outdoors and some people love to be in the gym. If you are going to stick with exercise it must be fun! Don't forget the E in FITTE.

> Have fun! Find your own way to help you stay active.

Involve Your Friends and Family. Exercising with other people is great. It builds commitment and keeps us motivated. You can encourage each other; when you're low on enthusiasm they won't be and when they are, you won't be. Use you heart attack as a reason to get your family and friends active, too. Be a role model to your children. You can inspire each other.

> *My half marathon time is faster than my grandson's! I'm 67, he is 27.*
>
> Bobby, age 67

When you're busy with family and work commitments it is easy to give up hobbies and social activities. Whether you're retired or still working, use exercise to be more sociable again; you'll be amazed at how much confidence it gives you.

Don't Get Bored. Having a regular balanced exercise programme is not only important for fitness but it stops you from getting bored (see chapter 5). Another way to reduce boredom and keep your body stimulated is to change your activity regularly. Maybe change with the season; try outside activities in the summer and indoor in the winter. Try new things.

Make It a Habit. Whatever exercise you choose to do regularly, get into a routine; make it a habit. Just vary what type of exercise you do so you don't get bored (see chapter 5).

Go Walking. Walking is a great way to be active. Strolling is better than nothing but to get the best effects, walk briskly. Brisk pace is different to everyone; it depends on your fitness and ability. Imagine you are late to meet a friend and need to go quickly. But remember, always start slowly and finish slowly. Listen to your body; it will tell you what brisk is.

Remember to wear good shoes and to walk in a tall, upright posture. Don't slouch. Pull in your tummy; you burn more calories this way. Do it like you mean it!

Leave the Car.   Get out of the habit of jumping in the car for short trips. Park your car a bit away from the shops and walk the last bit. Maybe you can walk the whole way, building it up gradually. Do as much as you can. Try to use public transport. This means you have to walk a bit at the beginning and at the end of your journey.

Join a Walking Group.   Walking on your own can be very relaxing, especially in the country or a park. Walking with other people is great fun, too, and some people feel safer when they are with others. If you join a walking group a group leader will plan the route. You might fancy an even bigger challenge. Hill walking introduces a higher-intensity of walking. But just like any exercise you must build it up gradually. It's a good idea to start on flatter walks especially if you have hip or knee problems. This is often called low-level walking or rambling. Some people use walking poles, which help take some of the load off the knees and hips and this way you're using your upper body so you're getting a whole-body workout. There are many local and national walking organisations. Try looking in your doctor's surgery, leisure centre, library and physiotherapy department. Or do a search on the Internet. Here are some good websites to start with:

www.walkit.com

www.activescotland.org

Wear a Pedometer.   Pedometers are great fun. They record the number of steps or miles you have walked. This is a great prompt to get you doing more and it's great reinforcement of how well you are doing. Pedometers can be inexpensive and getting feedback on your walking helps you to monitor your improvement.

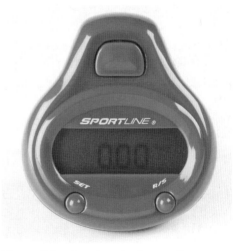

To start, aim for

3,500 to 5,500 a day if you are inactive or have been unwell.

6,000 to 8,500 a day if you are a healthy and active older adult.

9,000 to 13,000 a day if you are a healthy and active younger adult.

Once you are comfortably achieving your starting goal, then keep going and gradually add more steps.

Figure 8.1   A pedometer is a small, easy way to keep a real-time record of daily activity.

Keep a record of your steps so you can total up each week (see table 8.4). Remember to set a stepping goal that is realistic.

TABLE 8.4   **Keep Motivated by Recording Your Daily Total of Steps and Feelings**

Date	Number of steps	Comments
01/07	3,555	Felt great. Weather was lovely. Saw some deer in the park.
02/07	5,068	Walked with Beth. We had great chat!
03/07	4,445	Went to shopping mall at Goldenburn. Saw lots of other friends walking!
04/07	5,784	Walked with local ramblers on old canal; it was lovely. Saw ducks!

Go Shopping.   In the winter, when the weather is bad and it's dark by 5 p.m., try going to your local indoor shopping centre or mall. This lets you walk in a pleasant and safe environment. Take a friend to make it more fun and you can stop each other from buying things you don't need. Don't take your bankcard!

Get a Pet.   Walking is easy for people with a dog; you must have a routine.

Be Active on Your Holiday.   There are so many fun things to do such as walking, bowling, dancing, cycling, swimming, sailing, canoeing or archery. Challenge yourself and your family and friends. Try new things.

Water Exercise.   Water-based exercise might be a good option for you. People with painful hips, knees or back often find water-based exercise less painful. You could do some water-based exercise and some on the dry land every week; it's best to do a little bit of both. If you've recently had a heart event build up your fitness on the dry land for a while before exercising in the water and always check with your doctor or cardiac rehabilitation professional first before exercising in the water. Aqua fitness is a great way to exercise. You don't need to put your face in the water, you have the support of the water and you can have a good workout.

Top Tips for Sticking to a Healthy Diet

Think SMART.   Once you have decided to make changes to your diet, plan small changes that are realistic, that can be easily achieved and are relevant to you. These small changes can add up and become healthy habits over time, transforming your diet into a healthy one (refer to table 6.1).

Plan Your Meals.   You can plan by the week or even monthly if you are very organised. Try to plan at least 3 home-cooked meals a week (see recipes in appendix C), cook in batches and freeze meals in individual portioned containers to providing yourself with your own homemade ready meals at a fraction of the cost of eating out. Make use of your store cupboard essentials (see appendix D) such as pasta and tomato sauce. Add some frozen vegetables and you have a quick and easy delicious meal in minutes. Make a shopping list and stick to it to avoid unhealthy impulse buys. Shopping will be much quicker and you may even save some pennies.

Get Your Family on Board.   Let them know why you are making changes and encourage them to support you and make them too. Include them when planning and preparing meals. Plan meal times and try to eat with others as often as possible. This has lots of social and emotional benefits and can also help young children adopt healthy habits, too. The more support and encouragement you have, the more likely you are to stick with your new habits.

Pay Attention to Portions.   Most people have been brought up to finish what's on their plate but sometimes it is more than they really need. It is easy to eat too much, especially when larger-than-recommended portions are readily available. Try to aim for one third of your plate to be vegetables or try using a smaller plate at home to make it feel like you have more food on your plate.

Take Your Time.   Take time to chew and enjoy your food. It takes around 20 minutes for your body to register you are full, so fast eaters tend to eat more than their bodies need. Try not to do anything else when eating so you can learn to get more pleasure and satisfaction from your food.

Remember the Eatwell Plate.   The eatwell plate shows a healthy, balanced diet containing a wide variety of foods. Try something new each week and remember that no foods are off limits; all can be enjoyed in moderation.

This may be the end of the book, but it is the start of your journey. We hope this book has answered many of your questions and dispelled the common myths surrounding heart ill-health. You can now move forward confidently and know that there is a bright future. This book can be revisited at any time to help support you and those closest to you. Whether you are trying to make changes to one or many areas of your lifestyle, remember small changes make a big difference over time. The more positive changes you make, the more confident and good about yourself you will feel. In turn, the better you feel, the more likely you are to stick with the changes. You've reached the end of the book, but this is the start of your journey towards a healthy lifestyle and healthy heart.

Now it's time for you to take control.

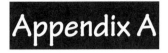

Templates for Helping You Plan

The following forms can be found at www.HumanKinetics.com/products/all-products/Healthy-Heart-Book-The

Planning Your Activity:
Sit Less, Move More

I, _____ , will sit for shorter periods in the following ways:

1._____

2._____

3._____

4._____

Witness _____ Date _____

From M. Thow, K. Graham, and C. Lee, 2013, *The healthy heart book* (Champaign, IL: Human Kinetics).

Planning Your Activity:
Accumulate 30 Minutes

I, _____ , will accumulate 30 minutes of activity every day in the following ways:

1._____

2._____

3._____

4._____

Witness _____ Date _____

From M. Thow, K. Graham, and C. Lee, 2013, *The healthy heart book* (Champaign, IL: Human Kinetics).

Planning Your Regular Exercise

I, _____, will do this structured exercise:

1._____

starting on _____ with _____.

2._____

starting on _____ with _____.

3._____

starting on _____ with _____.

4._____

starting on _____ with _____.

Witness _____ Date _____

From M. Thow, K. Graham, and C. Lee, 2013, *The healthy heart book* (Champaign, IL: Human Kinetics).

Coping With Stress

Things that are distressing me:

1. _____

2. _____

3. _____

4. _____

Making a plan—things that will help me:

1. _____

2. _____

3. _____

4. _____

From M. Thow, K. Graham, and C. Lee, 2013, *The healthy heart book* (Champaign, IL: Human Kinetics).

Changing a Behaviour

I want to _____

Pros: _____

_____

_____

Cons: _____

_____

_____

From M. Thow, K. Graham, and C. Lee, 2013, *The healthy heart book* (Champaign, IL: Human Kinetics).

How to Be Active and Fit Forever

Goal: I want to be active and fit.

Ask yourself the following questions (even better, write down your answers):

1. Why do I want to be fit? _____
   _____
   _____
   _____

2. What activity have I enjoyed in the past? _____
   _____
   _____
   _____

3. What activity and exercise can I see myself doing now? When will I do it? Whom will I do it with? (Phone them. Make it definite, such as a specific day and time. Remember, don't try to do too much too soon; add one new thing at a time.) _____
   _____
   _____
   _____

4. What things might stop me—weather, money, busy at work, busy with family?
   _____
   _____
   _____
   _____

5. What will I do when I'm out of my usual routine? _____
   _____
   _____
   _____

6. How will I reward myself for my efforts? _____
   _____
   _____
   _____

From M. Thow, K. Graham, and C. Lee, 2013, *The healthy heart book* (Champaign, IL: Human Kinetics).

Appendix B

Healthy Food Swaps

It is easier to start with what you already eat and make minor changes because gradual changes are easier to accept. Try these easy food swaps to reduce saturated fat and calories in your diet.

When eaten	Instead of	Try this	Calories (kcal) saved	Saturated fat saved
Breakfast	Sugar puffs (50 g) made with whole milk (100 ml)	Porridge oats (50 g) made with water and semi-skimmed milk (100 ml)	27	0.4
	Glass of pure orange juice (250 ml)	Glass of pure orange juice (150 ml)	47	0
	Mug of coffee made with 2 tsp sugar and whole milk (30 ml)	Mug of coffee made with artificial sweeteners and semi-skimmed milk (30 ml)	53	0.1
Mid-morning snack	Mug of tea made with 2 tsp sugar and whole milk (30 ml)	Mug of tea made with artificial sweeteners and semi-skimmed milk (30 ml)	53	0.1
	2 chocolate digestive biscuits	2 tea biscuits	84	4.2
Lunch	White bread roll (55 g) spread with butter (12 g)	Wholegrain roll with low-fat spread (10 g)	50	5
	Cheddar cheese (40 g)	Slice of turkey breast (35 g)	120	8
	Salt and vinegar crisps (34.5 g)	Side salad—lettuce, cherry tomatoes, cucumber, celery and cress (50 g)	165	1
	Sachet of tomato Cup-a-Soup	Cup of homemade red lentil soup (see recipe in appendix C)	40	1
	Can of cola (330 ml)	Can of diet cola (330 ml)	137	0

When eaten	Instead of	Try this	Calories (kcal) saved	Saturated fat saved
Mid-afternoon snack	Mug of tea made with 2 tsp sugar and whole milk (30 ml)	Mug of tea made with sweeteners and semi-skimmed milk (30 ml)	53	0.1
	Small apple pie	Handful of dried fruit and nuts (40 g)	72	2
Evening meal	Deep-fried fish in batter and deep fried chips	Healthy baked fish and chips, served with garden peas (see recipe in appendix C)	51	2
	2 scoops of ice cream	Fresh strawberries (80 g) served with low-fat natural yoghurt (50 g)	200	7.5
	Glass of whole milk (200 ml)	Glass of semi-skimmed milk (200 ml)	30	3
Supper	2 slices of white bread toasted and spread with butter (20 g) and jam (20 g)	2 slice of wholemeal toast with low-fat spread (20 g)	23	8
	Sachet of hot chocolate (56 g) made with whole milk (200 ml)	Mug of peppermint tea	248	0
Total	3,426 kcal	1,973 kcal	1,453 kcal	42.4 g
	65 g saturated fat	15.6 g saturated fat		

Note: The healthy days eating plan is based on guideline daily amounts (GDAs) 2,000 kcal, 20 g saturated fat, 90 g sugar and 6 g salt each day for an average woman of normal, healthy weight. All calorie values are approximate and taken from a leading supermarket website.

Appendix C

Healthy Recipes

Carrot and Butter Bean Soup

Serves: 4
Preparation time: 15 minutes
Cook time: 40 minutes

Ingredients

3 medium-sized carrots, peeled and sliced

2 tsp or 10 ml vegetable oil

900 ml or 1 1/2 pints chicken or vegetable stock

150ml or 1/4 pint semi-skimmed milk

1 onion, peeled and finely chopped

1 small tin butter beans

1 tablespoon cornflour

Chopped fresh parsley

Method

1. Cook carrots and onions in sunflower oil to soften, add stock and simmer for 30 minutes.
2. Blend using a hand blender or mash until desired consistency.
3. Mix the cornflour with milk and add to soup, bring back to boil, stirring all the time.
4. Drain butter beans and add to soup; simmer for a few minutes.
5. Serve garnished with chopped parsley and serve with crusty bread.

Red Lentil Soup

Serves: 2
Preparation time: 15 minutes
Cook time: 30 minutes

Ingredients

2 large carrots, peeled and diced

1 medium onion, peeled and diced

4 heaped tbsp or 50 g red split lentils

568 ml or 1 pint chicken or vegetable stock

Chopped parsley to garnish

Method

1. Place the carrots, onion and stock in a pot

2. Bring to the boil and stir in the lentils; reduce the heat and simmer for approximately 30 minutes or until vegetables are tender.

3. Serve garnished with chopped parsley and serve with crusty bread.

Tomato and Basil Bruschetta

Serves: 1
Preparation time: 10 minutes
Cook time: 5 minutes

Ingredients

1 ciabatta roll, cut in half length ways

1 clove garlic, peeled and cut in half

1 tbsp or 15 ml olive oil

2 ripe plum tomatoes

Handful of fresh basil leaves

Black pepper

Method

1. Dice tomatoes and place in a large bowl.

2. Stir in olive oil, add basil leaves and add black pepper to taste; set aside.

3. Toast ciabatta on both sides and rub cut side with garlic.

4. Spoon tomato mixture over ciabatta, add black pepper to taste and serve immediately.

Salmon, Leek and Red Pepper Frittata

Serves: 4
Preparation time: 15 minutes
Cook time: 20 minutes

Ingredients

200 g or 8 oz cooked new potatoes

2 tbsp or 30 ml rapeseed oil

4 large eggs, beaten

1 medium red pepper, de-seeded and sliced

1 medium leek, trimmed and finely sliced

Dry or fresh parsley

1 medium tin salmon, drained and flaked

Black pepper to season

Method

1. Slice potatoes into thin disks.
2. Heat oil in a 22 cm non-stick frying pan. Add potatoes, peppers and leeks; cook for 5 minutes until soft and golden in colour.
3. Mix eggs with parsley and season with black pepper.
4. Add salmon flakes to pan and pour over egg mixture. Cook on a low heat for 5 minutes or until frittata is just set. Finish under a hot grill until firm and golden in colour.
5. Cut into 4 portions and serve each with a slice of crusty wholemeal bread and a large side salad.

Quick-Cooking Chicken Casserole

Serves: 4
Preparation time: 15 minutes
Cook time: 35 minutes

Ingredients

1 tbsp or 15 ml rapeseed oil

4 skinless chicken quarters or 4 small chicken breasts

1 red onion, peeled and chopped

1 clove garlic, peeled and crushed

1 red pepper, de-seeded and thickly sliced

2 tsp or 10 ml ground paprika

300 ml or 1/2 pint chicken stock

3 tbsp or 45 ml tomato puree

Black pepper to taste

Method

1. Heat oil in a large frying pan and fry chicken on all sides for 5 to 6 minutes or until golden brown (quarters will take longer than breasts). Lift out and discard oil.
2. Wipe the pan with a kitchen towel and heat remaining oil and fry garlic, onions and peppers for 3 to 4 minutes.
3. Return the chicken to the pan. Sprinkle over paprika and pour in stock.
4. Add the tomato puree and season with black pepper; bring to a boil.
5. Reduce heat and simmer for 20 minutes or until chicken is cooked through.
6. Serve with freshly cooked rice or potatoes and plenty of vegetables on the side.

Tasty Oven Fish and Chips

Serves: 2
Preparation time: 15 minutes
Cook time: 30 minutes

Ingredients

2 150 g or 2 6 oz-thick cod steaks

2 slices granary or wholewheat bread made into breadcrumbs

1 small egg, beaten

Black pepper to taste

2 wedges fresh lemon to garnish

Method

1. Preheat oven to 200°C (400°C, gas mark 6)
2. Toast or brown breadcrumbs on a non-stick baking tray in oven for 10 minutes.
3. Place egg on a shallow plate and season fish with black pepper on both sides. Dip fish into egg on both sides and coat in breadcrumbs.
4. Place on non-stick baking tray in centre of oven for 20 minutes or until golden and cooked through.
5. Serve with homemade oven chips, peas and a wedge of fresh lemon

Note: To make breadcrumbs place bread in a food processor and blend to desired consistency or use a grater. Day-old bread works best.

Homemade Oven Chips

Serves: 2
Preparation time: 10 minutes
Cook time: 40 minutes

Ingredients

360 g or 2 medium-sized potatoes, washed with skins left on

2 tbsp or 30 ml olive oil

Black pepper to taste

Method

1. Preheat oven to 200°C (400°C, gas mark 6)
2. Scrub the potatoes and cut them into thick, chunky chips.
3. Boil for 5 minutes, drain water and add olive oil giving pan a good shake to coat chips in oil.
4. Spread onto a pre-heated non stick baking tray, season with black pepper and bake on top shelf of oven for 30 minutes.

For a variation sprinkle 1 or 2 tsp chilli or curry powder over the chips before coating in the oil.

Penne Arrabiata

Serves: 2
Preparation time: 5 minutes
Cook time: 12 minutes

Ingredients

150 g or 6 oz dry penne pasta

1 tsp or 5 ml olive oil

1 garlic clove, peeled and chopped

1 small chilli, de-seeded and sliced thinly

Handful of fresh basil leaves

400 g or 16 oz tin chopped tomatoes

2 tbsp or 30 g grated parmesan cheese

Black pepper

Method

1. Heat the oil in a non-stick frying pan and add the garlic and chilli. After 1 minute add the basil leaves into the oil mixture.

2. Remove the mixture from pan and set aside, add chopped tomatoes and add chilli mixture back to pan. Simmer for 10 minutes.

3. Meanwhile, cook pasta to pack instructions in a large pan of boiling water.

4. Drain the pasta and add to the tomato sauce mixture.

5. Serve with a sprinkle of the grated parmesan cheese and black pepper to taste.

Chilli Con Carne

Serves: 4
Preparation time: 15 minutes
Cook time: 30 minutes

Ingredients

1 large onion, peeled and finely chopped

1 red or green pepper, de-seeded and finely chopped

2 tsp or 10 ml rapeseed oil

200 g or 8oz extra lean minced beef

400 g or 16 oz tin chopped tomatoes and herbs

200 g or 8 oz tin red kidney beans, drained

200 g or 8 oz long grain rice

1 or 2 cloves garlic, peeled and finely chopped

1 tbsp or 15 ml tomato puree

1 tsp or 5 ml chilli powder

Method

1. Dry-fry the mince in a non-stick pan until brown, remove from pan and keep warm.

2. Heat the oil in the pan and fry onion and peppers for 3 minutes or until soft.

3. Add the garlic and fry for 30 seconds.

4. Add the browned mince and chilli powder, stir and mix well.

5. Stir in tomatoes, kidney beans and tomato puree. Bring to the boil and simmer for 20 minutes.

6. Serve with plain boiled rice.

Oven-Baked Chocolate Banana

Serves: 2
Preparation time: 5 minutes
Cook time: 20-30 minutes

Ingredients

2 medium-sized ripe bananas

12 chocolate buttons

Natural yoghurt to serve (optional)

Method

1. Keeping the skin on the bananas and using a sharp knife, slice each banana lengthways carefully leaving the bottom of the skin intact.

2. Insert 6 chocolate buttons along each opening and wrap the bananas individually in silver foil.

3. Bake in the oven for 20 to 30 minutes until bananas are soft and the chocolate has melted.

4. Remove bananas from the foil and skin

5. Serve with a few spoons natural yoghurt (optional).

Easy Fruit Jelly

Serves: 4
Preparation time: 5 minutes
Chill time: approximately 3-4 hours

Ingredients

1 packet strawberry or raspberry sugar-free jelly

300 g or 12 oz mixed fresh, frozen or tinned berries in fruit juice (strawberries, raspberries or blackberries)

Method

1. Dissolve jelly as per pack instructions; if using tinned fruit some of the fruit juice can be used instead of the cold water to make up jelly.

2. Pour into a large jelly mould or 4 individual dishes. Place in refrigerator until partially set.

3. Add the fruit and return to refrigerator until fully set.

Note: Allowing the jelly to partially set before adding fruit stops the fruit falling to the bottom. The fruit can be added once you have poured the jelly in to the moulds if you would rather not wait.

Store Cupboard, Fridge and Freezer Essentials

Some of the healthy recipes include basic store cupboard essentials, which can usually be stored for a long time. Here are a few ideas to get you started. Choose what you like and gradually build up your stocks.

Bread, Rice, Potatoes, Pasta and Other Starches

Pasta such as macaroni, spaghetti and penne; try whole-wheat varieties

Egg or rice noodles

Rice such as brown, long-grain, basmati or Arborio

Couscous

Breads such as tortilla wraps and pitta bread: try wholemeal varieties

Flour such as white, wholemeal or cornflour

Fruit and Vegetables

Tinned fruit such as mandarin oranges, fruit cocktail or pineapple chunks in juice

Pure fruit juice with no added sugar: apple, orange, tomato or pineapple

Frozen mixed berries

Tinned vegetables such as peas, carrots, sweetcorn and tomatoes

Frozen vegetables such as peas, green beans, broccoli and cauliflower

Meat, Fish, Eggs and Beans

Small or medium eggs

Tinned fish such as salmon, sardines, mackerel and tuna: try for varieties in tomato sauce, sunflower oil, olive oil or spring water

Frozen fish such as salmon, trout and kippers

Pulses such as lentils, chick peas, kidney beans, butter beans and broth mix

Milk and Dairy Foods

UHT long-life milk

Low-fat natural yoghurt

Low-fat crème fraîche

Low-fat cottage cheese

Condiments, Oils, Vinegars, Spices and Herbs

    Olive oil, rapeseed oil, vegetable oil

    Low-fat spread

    Balsamic vinegar

    White wine vinegar

    Tomato puree, mustard, Worcestershire sauce

    Stock cubes such as vegetable, chicken, ham or beef

    Curry powder or paste

    Chilli powder or sauce

    Ground paprika

    Black pepper

    Mixed herbs

    Oregano

    Parsley

    Rosemary

    Thyme

Appendix E

Exercise Programme

Which Exercise Programme Do I Choose?

Before you begin an exercise programme, you need to choose the one that is appropriate for you:

1. If you have problems with balance, choose programme 1 (light t-shirt).
2. If you have no balance problems, choose programme 2 (dark t-shirt).

Once you have chosen the appropriate programme, keep in mind the following:

- The exercise programmes are designed to include a warm-up, workout, and cool-down. Always follow the exercises in the order advised.
- The warm-up and cool-down should feel light, so do them slowly.
- For the workout, move at a speed that feels comfortable. Take it gently the first time you do the exercises. You can speed up as you get used to the programme and as you become fitter and more confident.
- During the workout your exertion level should be between 4 and 6 (see the exertion scale at the end of this appendix). Keep your exertion levels on the lower side to begin with (4-5). After a few weeks of doing the workout regularly, then increase your level to 6. To revise how to use the exertion scale, see chapter 4.
- Make sure that it is safe to exercise by revising the section 'Keep It Safe' in chapter 5.
- If you have been having angina symptoms, revise 'What to do if You Think You Are Having Angina' in chapter 1.

Starting Your Programme

- Copy or cut out the exertion scale at the end of this appendix and stick it up on the wall at eye level so that you can see it easily. Look at the exertion scale and think about how you are feeling whilst you are exercising.
- Copy or cut out the exercises and stick your exercise programme up on the wall next to your exertion scale.

Each time you are ready to begin your programme, do the following:

- Prepare the area. Clear some space so you have plenty of room to move.
- Exercise in a room with a window and open it if you get too warm.
- Wear loose, comfortable clothing that allows you to move freely.
- Wear supportive, flat shoes (trainers if you have them).
- Keep hydrated. Have a glass of water ready and have a drink every so often whilst you are exercising.
- Put on some music. Nothing too fast, just something fun, uplifting and motivating.

Making Progress

If you notice the exercise is getting too easy for you, you have three choices for making it more challenging. During the workout portion of your exercise programme, you can do one or more of the following:

1. Increase the time you spend on each exercise; see advice within each programme.
2. Move faster and make your steps bigger.
3. Have a small hand weight in each hand or use a small water bottle. Empty the water out and take the label off so it is easy to grip. Fill the bottle with rice, lentils, sand or stones and weigh it (a kitchen scale is helpful). Start with 0.5 kg (1 lb), then increase to 1 kg (2 lb) and then increase to 1.5 kg (3 lb). Remember not to use hand weights during your warm-up or cool-down.

Programme 1

This programme should take 30 to 45 minutes. You need your two small bottles of water or small hand weights for the workout portion of this exercise programme.

Do the exercises in this order:

1 to 8

1 to 8 again

9 to 12

9 to 12 again

13 to 24

13 to 24 again

12 to 1 (reverse)

25 to 30

When the exercise programme starts to feel too easy, try one of the following:

- Add a third set of repetitions 13 to 24.
- Increase the time you spend on exercises 13 to 24 to 1 minute.

Warm-Up

- Sit in an upright chair (no arms on chair).
- Keep good posture. Try not to lean back in the chair. Sit up straight, pulling in your abdominal muscles. If you need to lean back in the chair and have a rest at points throughout the programme then do so and then sit up straight again as soon as you can.
- Start with your feet on the floor at hip-distance apart and your hands facing palms down on your thighs.

Perform each exercise 10 times.

1. **Look over one shoulder**—5 times to the left and centre followed by 5 times to the right and centre.
2. **Toe taps**—Tap your toes up and down.

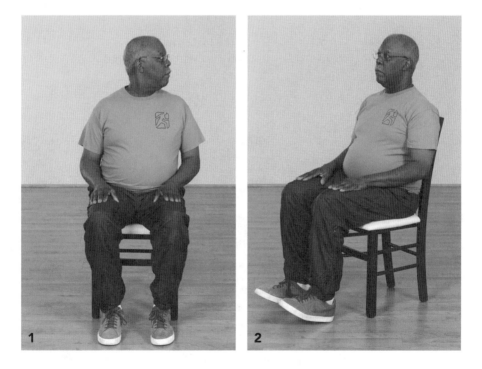

3. **Ankle circles**—Circle your left ankle 5 times each way, then circle the right ankle 5 times each way.

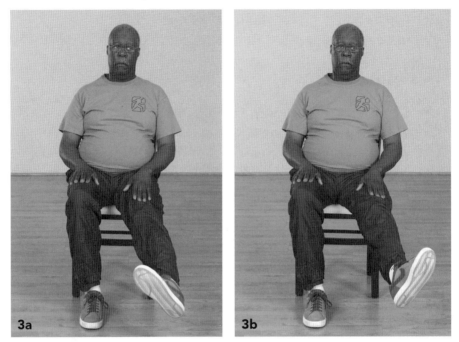

4. **Heel digs**—Tap your left heel in front, then back to where it started. Tap your right heel in front then back to where it started. Continue alternating from left to right.

5. **Marching**—March your feet on the spot; step right, left, right, left, and so on.

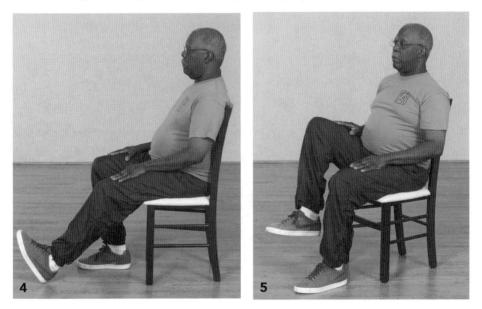

6. **Heel raises**—Lift both heels firmly up and down.

7. **Side taps**—Tap the left foot to the side, then bring it back to where it started. Tap the right foot to the side, then back to where it started. Continue, alternating left and right.

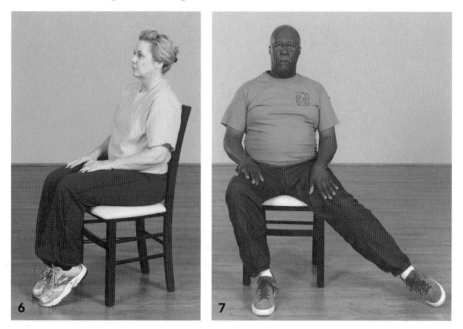

8. **Knee extensions**—Straighten the left knee, then place it back to where it started. Straighten the right knee, then bring it back to where it started. Try to make your knee is completely straight each time. Continue alternating.

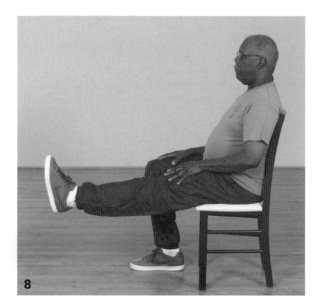

9. **Toe taps with shoulder shrugs**—Do toe taps as before whilst shrugging the shoulders up and down.

10. **Heel digs with biceps curls**—Do heel digs as before whilst bending and straightening the elbows.

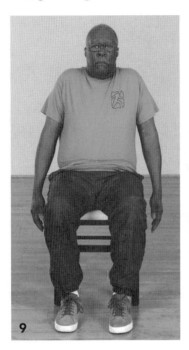 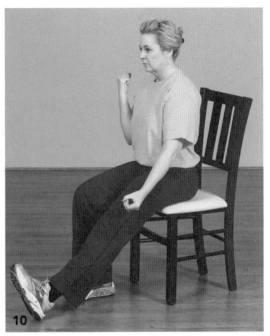

11. **Heel raises with punching forwards**—Do heel raises as before whilst punching the arms forwards and back.

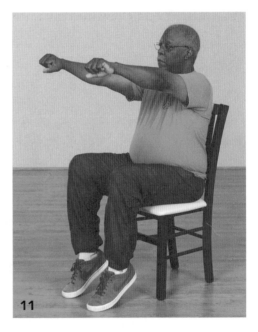

12. **Side taps with side punches**—Do side taps as before whilst punching to the sides.

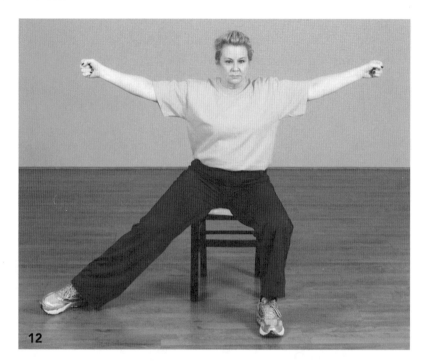

Workout

- Stand up. Keep your chair in front of you so you can lean on it for balance. Use a chair that is high enough so that you are not leaning forwards. You could use a table, a window ledge or the kitchen work surface.
- Keep good posture. Stand up tall, pulling in your abdominal muscles.
- To start, do exercises 16, 20 and 24 sitting down. As the programme starts to feel easier you can stand up for these three exercises and march on the spot whilst lifting the water bottles or small weights.

Perform each exercise for 30 seconds.

13. **Heel raises**—Go up and down on your tiptoes. Do both feet together. Do this slowly and controlled.

14. **Kickbacks**—Kick a heel back and up towards your bottom. Continue, alternating left and right.

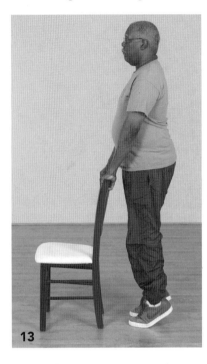 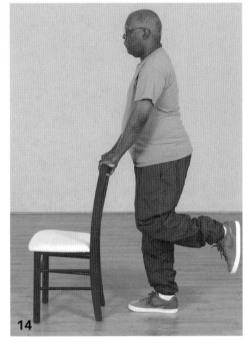

15. **Side taps**—Tap your toe to one side, then back to the start position. Continue, alternating left and right.

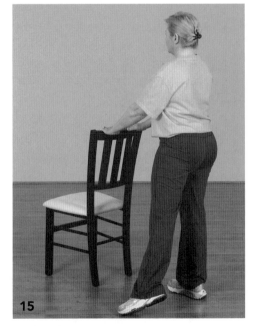

16. **Sit down**—Do heel digs with biceps curls (small water bottle or weights in both hands).

17. **Marching on the spot**—March your feet, alternately lifting them up and down on the spot.

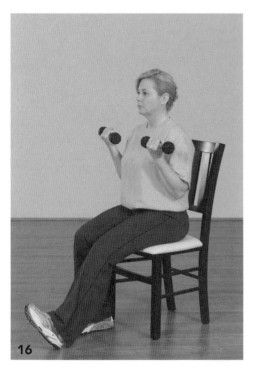

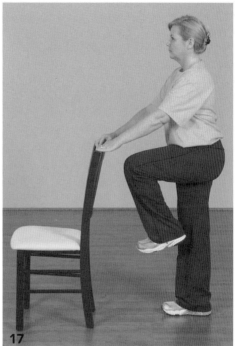

18. **Tap backs**—Tap one foot behind you, then return it to start position. Continue, alternating left and right.

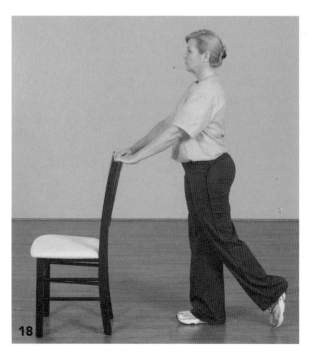

19. **Side taps**—Tap your toe to the side, then back to the start position. Continue, alternating left and right.

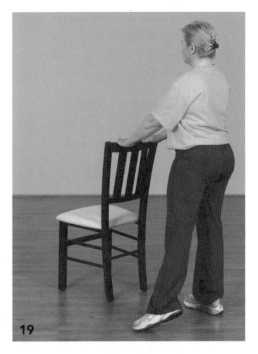

20. **Sit down**—Do a side tap with punches to the side (small water bottles or weights in both hands).

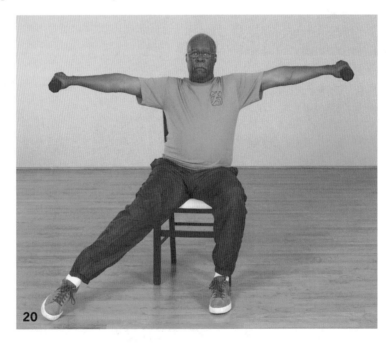

21. **Minisquats**—Stick your bottom out and bend your knees, keeping your heels on the floor. Stand up again.

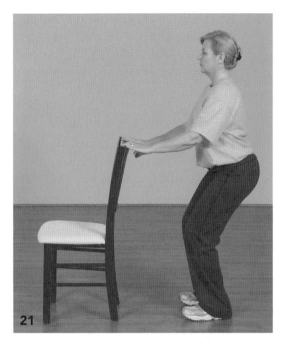

22. **Wall press**—This is like a press-up against the wall. Stand facing the wall. Put your hands on the wall at shoulder height. Bend and straighten the elbows. As you do this exercise, keep pulling in your abdominal muscles and keep your back straight. To make it harder, take your feet further away from the wall.

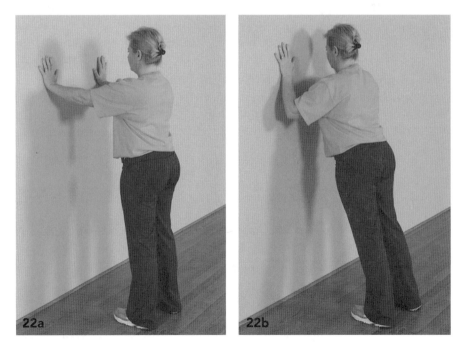

23. **Sit to stand**—Come to the edge of the chair. Stand up tall, making sure the backs of your knees are touching the chair, then sit back down. To make it easier, push up using your hands on your thighs; to make it harder, don't use your hands to push up.

24. **Sit down**—Do toe taps while punching forwards (small water bottle or weights in both hands)

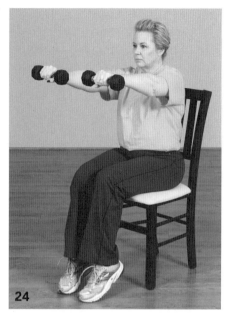

24

Cool-Down

Do the opposite of the warm-up; do exercises 12 to 1 in reverse order.

Stretches:

* Hold each stretch for 15 to 20 seconds.
* Don't hold your breath. Breathe slowly and deeply as you stretch; this helps your muscles to relax.
* Go as far as you can with each stretch. It should not be painful but you should feel slight discomfort.

25. **Upper back**—Make a circle with your arms. Push your hands away from your body and tuck your chin in a little.

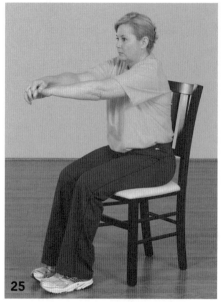

25

26. **Chest**—Put the palms of your hands into the small of your back and squeeze your elbows back. If you have a chest wound start this stretch 5 weeks after your surgery. This is still a good stretch to do, build up gradually; don't force it.

27. **Shoulders**—Reach across your body. Use your other hand to press over into a stretch.

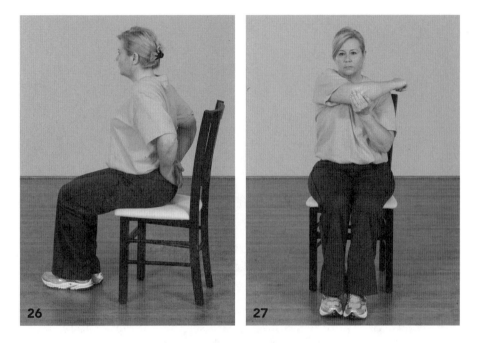

28. **Hamstrings**—Sit nearer the edge of the chair so that you can put your heel on the floor with your leg straight. Put your hands on the opposite leg for balance. Keep your body straight and lean forwards from your hips. Pull your toes up. Then do the same to the opposite side.

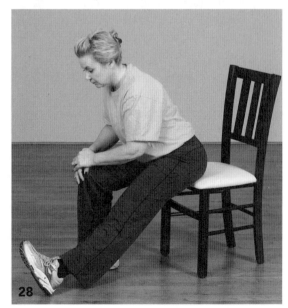

29. **Trunk**—Put your left hand on your left hip and your right hand on your right shoulder. Lean to your left and bring your right elbow up as far as you can. Don't lean forwards. Then do the same to the opposite side.

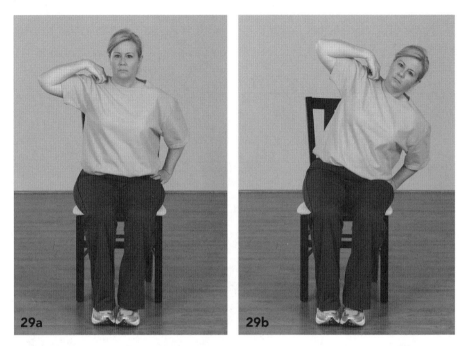

30. **Deep breathing for relaxation**—Place your hands on your abdomen. Relax your shoulders. Soften the muscles in your face (no tension in your forehead or around your eyes). Take a long, slow breath in followed by a longer, slower breath out. Count up to 3 slowly as you breathe in. Count up to 4 slowly as you breathe out. Do this 10 times. (For more detail on deep breathing, see chapter 7.)

Programme 2

This programme should take 45 to 60 minutes.

Do the exercises in this order:

1 to 7 (30 seconds each)

8 to 14—single arm, alternating left and right arms (30 seconds each)

8 to 14—double arms, both arms at the same time (30 seconds each)

15 to 26—1 minute each

15 to 26—1 minute each

14 to 1 (reverse)

27 to 35

When the exercise programme starts to feel too easy, try one of the following:

- Increase the amount of time you spend doing exercises 15 to 26 to 1 minute and 30 seconds.
- Use your small water bottle or weight in each hand when doing exercises 15, 17, 19, 21, 23, 25. It should not feel painful. Put the water bottle down if your arms are getting very tired.

Warm-Up

- Keep good posture. Stand up tall with you feet hip-distance apart and pull in your abdominal muscles.
- Control your movements. Place your feet softly when moving.

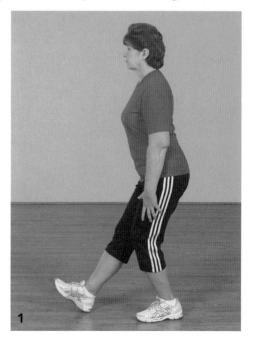

1. **Heel digs**—Tap your right heel in front, then back to where it started. Tap your left heel in front, then back to where it started. Continue, alternating right and left.

2. **Side taps**—Tap the right foot to the side, then bring it back to where it started. Tap the left foot to the side, then back to where it started. Continue, alternating right and left.

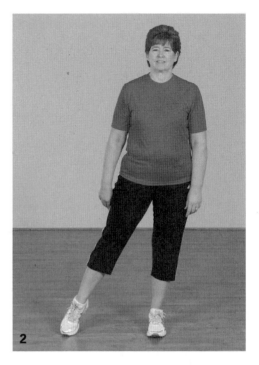

3. **Tap back**—Tap one foot behind you, then back to start position. Continue, alternating left and right.

4. **Side step**—Step to the right, then back to the middle. Step to the left, then back to middle. Continue, alternating left and right.

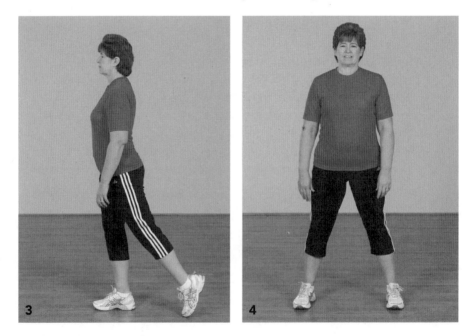

5. **Marching on the spot**—March left, right, left, right, and so on. Be light on your feet.

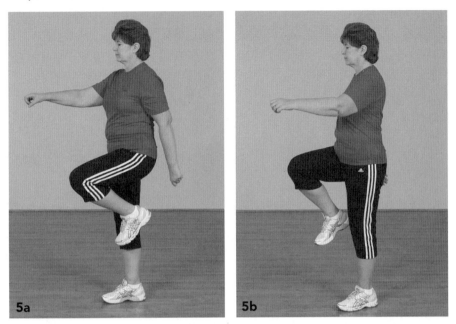

6. **Hamstring curls**—Start with your feet wide apart. Kick your left heel towards your right buttock, then your right heel towards your left buttock. Continue, alternating left and right.

7. **Knee lifts**—Raise your left knee up to hip height, then place it back down. Continue, alternating left and right.

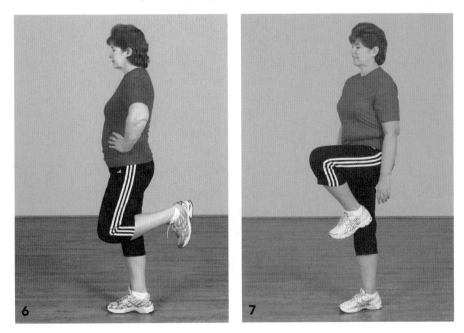

8. **Heel digs with biceps curls**—Do heel digs as before whilst bending one arm up, then the other.

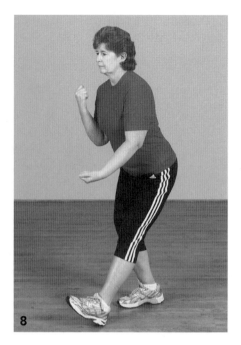

9. **Side taps with lateral raise**—Tap the right toes to the right and lift the arms to the sides, then come back to where you started. Continue, alternating left and right.

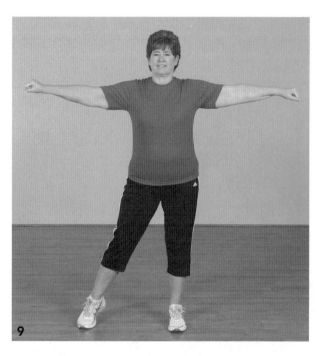

10. **Tap back with shoulder swing**—Tap back as before. Swing one arm upwards. Continue, alternating left and right.

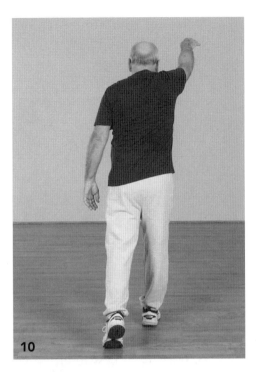

11. **Side step with side punch**—Side step as before. Punch your right hand to the side and then punch your left hand to the side. Continue, alternating right and left.

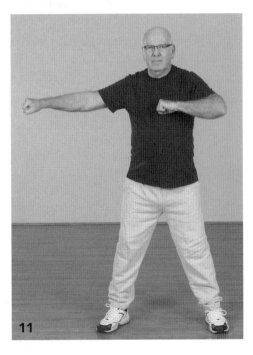

12. **Marching with arm swing—** Marching on the spot, swing the arms.

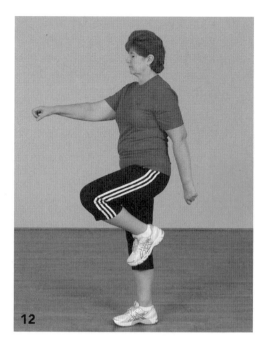

13. **Hamstring curls with upright row**—Do hamstring curls as before. Make fists with your hands and lift your hands up and down. Your elbows should come up to shoulder height (like zipping up a jacket).

14. **Knee lifts and tap hands to knee**—Lift the right knee up to hip height and tap your hands to your knee. Then lift the left knee and tap your hands to your knee. Continue, alternating left and right.

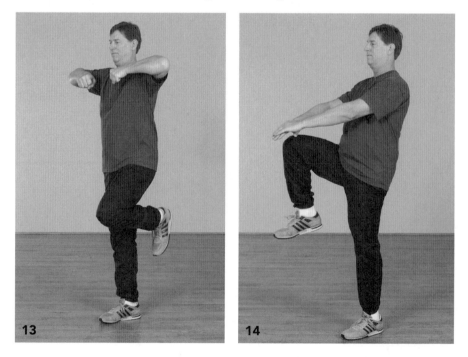

Workout

15. **Sit to stand**—Come to the edge of the chair, stand up tall, making sure the backs of your knees are touching the chair and sit back down. To make it harder, do not push up using your hands on your thighs and punch your hands forwards as you stand up.

16. **Side taps with double punch**—Do a side tap as before whilst punching both hands above your head.

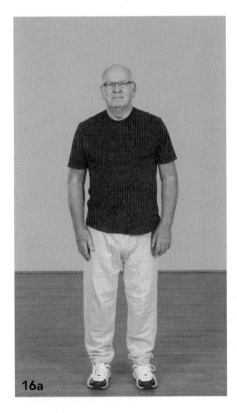
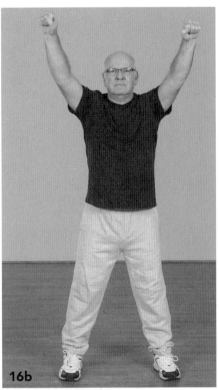

17. **Heel digs with high biceps curls**—Do heel digs as before, adding double biceps curls (both arms simultaneously) at shoulder height.

18. **Squats**—Stick your bottom out and bend your knees, keeping your heels on the floor. Stand up again. As you bend your knees punch your hands forwards.

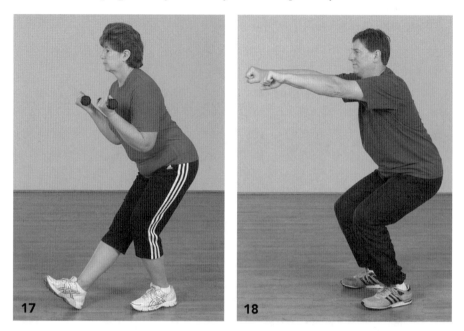

19. **Tap back with pec deck**—Tap back as before. Keeping the elbows bent and held at shoulder height, squeeze both elbows forwards and back.

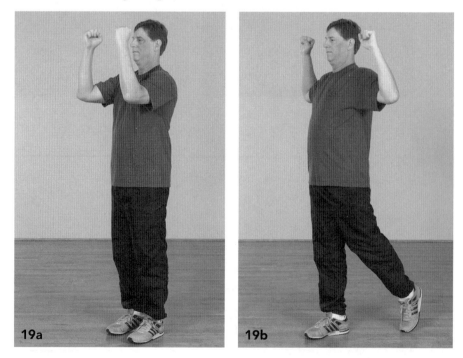

20. **Knee lifts with double punch upwards**—Do knee lifts as before whilst punching both hands above your head.

21. **Side steps with hands crossed**—Side step whilst crossing your hands behind your back.

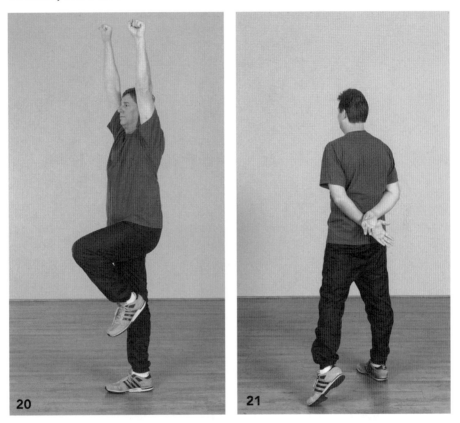

22. **Wall press**—This is the same as exercise 10 from programme 1. Stand facing the wall. Put your hands on the wall at shoulder height, then bend and straighten your elbows. As you do this exercise, keep pulling in your abdominal muscles and keep your back straight. To make this exercise harder, take your feet further away from the wall.

23. **Marching with rope climb**—Marching on the spot, pretend to climb a rope with your arms.

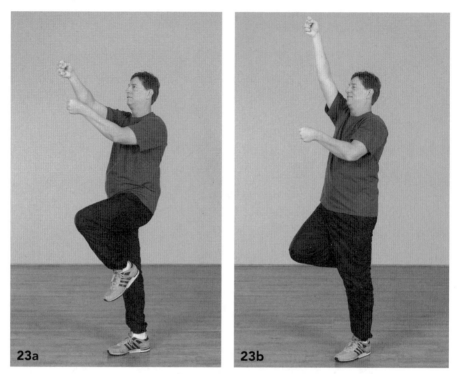

24. **Hamstring curls with lateral pull-backs**—Do hamstring curls whilst reaching forwards and pulling the elbows back. Squeeze the shoulder blades together.

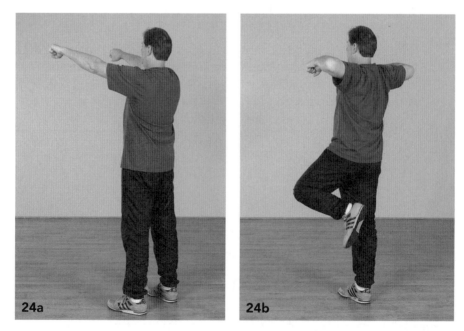

25. **Knee lifts with double punch**—Do knee lifts whilst punching both arms above your head.

26. **Heel raise with arm swing**—Do heel raises whilst swinging both arms up and forwards.

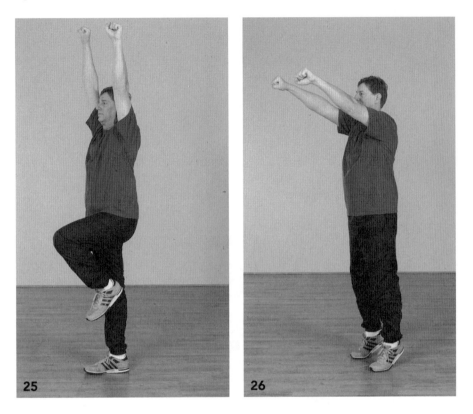

Cool-Down

Do the opposite of the warm-up; do exercises 14 to 1 in reverse order.

Stretches:

- Hold each stretch for 15 to 20 seconds.
- Don't hold your breath. Breathe slowly and deeply as you stretch; this helps your muscles to relax.
- Go as far as you can with each stretch. It should not be painful but you should feel slight discomfort.

27. **Shoulders**—Reach across your body and use your other hand to press over into a stretch. Keep your feet moving slowly with a small side step.

28. **Triceps**—Put your left hand on your left shoulder. Use your right hand to push the elbow up until you feel a stretch down the back of the upper arm. Now stretch the other arm.

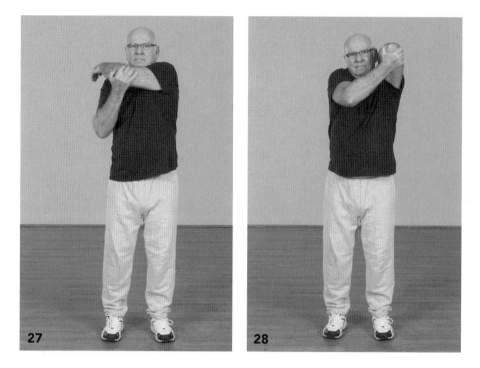

29. **Neck**—Look over your right shoulder. Look over your left shoulder. Keep your feet moving slowly with a small side step.

30. **Hamstrings**—Bend your knees. Take your weight onto one leg and put the other heel in front. Stick your bottom out. Put your hands on your bent leg for balance and lean forwards from your hips. Do the same stretch to the opposite side. Keep your arms moving with slow biceps curls so that you are gradually reducing the workload on your heart and not suddenly stopping. You want the blood to keep flowing.

31. **Calf**—Take a big step back with one leg. Keeping your back leg straight and your heel firmly on the ground, bend your front knee. Tip your body forwards a little. Do the same stretch to the opposite side. Keep your arms moving with shoulder shrugs.

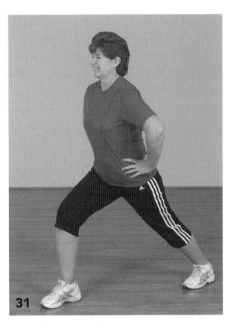

32. **Quadriceps**—Rest your hand on the wall for balance. Bend your left leg and use your left hand to hold onto your left foot, sock or trouser leg (whichever you can reach). Pull your heel toward your bottom. Make sure you stand up straight.

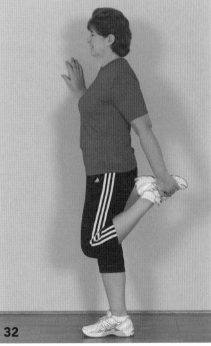

33. **Chest**—Put your hands into the small of your back and squeeze your elbows back. If you have a chest wound start this stretch 5 weeks after your surgery. This is still a good stretch to do, but don't force it; build up gradually.

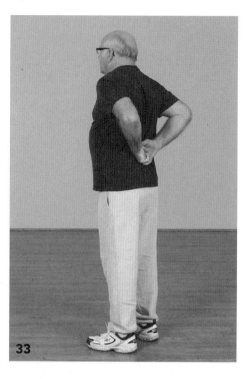

34. **Upper back and shoulder blades**—Make a circle with your arms. Push your hands away from your body and tuck your chin in a little.

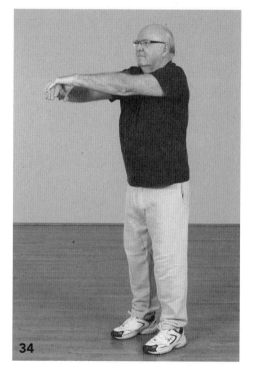

35. **Deep breathing for relaxation**—Place your hands on your abdomen. Relax your shoulders. Soften the muscles in your face (no tension in your forehead or around your eyes). Take a long slow breath in followed by a longer slower breath out. Count up to three slowly as you breathe in. Count up to four slowly as you breathe out. Do this 10 times. (For more detail on deep breathing, see chapter 7.)

THE EXERTION SCALE Listen to Your Body

	How much exertion?	How does it feel in your muscles and breathing?	The talk test
0	Complete rest	Relaxed breathing, relaxed muscles (sitting still)	You can sing and whistle whilst exerting yourself.
1	Minimum effort	Normal breathing, no muscle strain	
2	Extremely mild effort	Just aware of breathing more deeply, aware of very slight muscle strain	
3	Somewhat mild effort		
4	Mild effort	Breathing more deeply, muscles lightly strained	You can talk comfortably whilst exerting yourself.
5	Medium effort	Breathing deeply, definite muscle strain but comfortable, able to continue	
6	Fairly strenuous effort		
7	Strenuous effort	Breathing really deeply, muscles very strained, feeling like you would like to slow down	You are struggling to talk in sentences whilst exerting yourself, gasping for breath.
8	Very strenuous effort		
9	Extremely strenuous effort	The hardest effort you have ever felt; muscles and breathing are pushed to a very high level	
10	Maximum exertion	The maximal exertion that could possibly be achieved; most people will never feel this	

Useful Contacts
and Organisations

Alcohol Concern

64 Leman Street

London E1 8EU

Tel: 020 7264 0510

Website: www.alcoholconcern.org.uk

National alcohol charity working against alcohol misuse.

Alcoholics Anonymous (AA), UK headquarters

P.O. Box 1

10 Toft Green

York YO1 7NJ

Tel: 0190 464 4026

Alcoholics Anonymous (AA)

Scottish headquarters

Baltic Chambers

50 Wellington Street

Glasgow G2 6HJ

Tel: 0141 226 2214

Website: www.alcoholics-anonymous.org.uk

Worldwide charity that offers information and support through local groups to people with alcohol problems who want to stop drinking.

Action on Smoking and Health (ASH)

First Floor

144-145 Shoreditch High Street

London E1 6JE

Tel: 020 7739 5902

E-mail: enquiries@ash.org.uk

Website: www.ash.org.uk

National organisation with local branches offering free information on quitting smoking.

Blood Pressure Association

60 Cranmer Terrace

London W17 0QS

Tel: 020 8772 4994

Information Line: 0845 241 0989 (Mondays-Fridays, 11 a.m.-3 p.m.)

Website: www.bpassoc.org.uk

Provides information and advice regarding causes, treatment and advice for people living with high blood pressure.

British Association Cardiovascular Prevention and Rehabilitation (BACPR)

c/o BCS

9 Fitzroy Square

London W1T 5HW

Tel: 020 7380 1919

Website: www.bacpr.com

Registered charity that provides, develops and improves core standards to ensure the safe delivery of cardiovascular prevention and rehabilitation practice and programmes in the United Kingdom.

British Nutrition Foundation

High Holborn House

52-54 High Holborn

London WC1 6RQ

Tel: 020 7404 6504

Website: www.nutrition.org.uk

Provides evidence-based information on food and nutrition.

British Heart Foundation (BHF)

Greater London House

180 Hampstead Road

London NW1 7AW

Tel: 020 7554 0000

Heart help line: 0300 330 3311 (Mondays-Fridays, 9 a.m.-5 p.m.)

Website: www.bhf.org.uk

National charity that funds research, provides education and publishes a range of information on heart disease, lifestyle issues, tests and treatments and sympathetic insurance companies.

Chest Heart & Stroke Scotland (CHSS) Head Office

Third Floor

Rosebery House

Haymarket Terrace

Edinburgh EH12 5EZ

Tel: 0131 225 6963

Advice line: 0845 077 6000 (Monday–Friday, 9.30 a.m.-12.30 p.m., 1.30 p.m.-4 p.m.)

Website: www.chss.org.uk

Scottish charity that funds research in the prevention, diagnosis, treatment, rehabilitation and the social impact of chest, heart and stroke illness. They publish a range of information on heart disease, lifestyle issues, tests and treatments and sympathetic insurance companies

Diabetes UK

Central Office

Macleod House

10 Parkway

London NW1 7AA

Tel: 020 7424 1000

Website: www.diabetes.org.uk

National organisation with local groups that provides advice and information on diabetes.

electronic Medicines Compendium (eMC)

Website: www.medicines.org.uk

Provides up to date news and information about UK licensed medicines.

Food Standards Agency

Aviation House

125 Kingsway

London WC2B 6NH

Tel: 020 7276 8960

Website: www.food.gov.uk

UK Government body showing current research in food safety, nutrition and food-related disease.

Heart UK

The Cholesterol Charity

7 North Road

Maidenhead

Berkshire SL6 1PE

Helpline: 0845 450 5988 (Tuesdays and Thursdays 10 a.m.-4 p.m.)

Website: www.heartuk.org.uk

National charity that provides information and advice for people with high cholesterol levels.

NHS choices

Website www.nhs.uk

NHS Choices is the online 'front door' to the NHS. It is the country's biggest health website and gives all the information you need to make choices about your health.

Northern Ireland Chest Heart and Stroke

21 Dublin Road

Belfast

BT2 7HB

Tel: 02890320184

Website: www.nichsa.com

Northern Ireland charity that funds research in the prevention, diagnosis, treatment, rehabilitation and the social impact of chest, heart and stroke illness. Its main work is focused in four areas: research, advocacy and lobbying, health promotion and care services.

QUIT

63 St.Marys Axe

London EC3A 8AA

Tel: 0207 469 0400

Quitline—Tel: 0800 00 22 00.

Website: www.quit.org.uk

UK based charity that helps smokers to stop. This website provides help and advice for smokers, health professionals, employers and teachers.

SMOKEFREE

Tel: 0800 022 4 332

Website: www.smokefree.nhs.uk

Get free support, expert advice and tools including the Quit Kit to help you stop smoking. Watch videos from real quitters on what helped them stop.

The following websites will give you ideas and support with your ongoing activity and exercise.

www.walkit.com—The urban walking map and route planner that helps you get around town on foot. Get a walking route map between any two points, including your journey time.

www.activescotland.org—Provides help with finding activities local to your selected postcode.

www.ouractivenation.co.uk—Encourages people to take part in easy exercises, simple exercise to do at home and easy ways to get fit. It contains an activity finder and lots of links to other activities.

www.physicalactivityandnutritionwales.org.uk—Physical Activity and Nutrition network for Wales. Encourages activity and healthy eating

Information on Stress and Relaxation Techniques

The following websites provide self-help information on stress, including relaxation techniques. Some of these websites allow you to download audio or visual files demonstrating relaxation techniques on to your computer or MP3 player. Some also allow you to print off instructions on relaxation techniques. A range of relaxation techniques available. Breathing techniques and PMR are good places to start, but experiment to see what suits you.

www.mentalhealth.org.uk/information/wellbeing-podcasts—A range of podcasts containing music and relaxation instructions.

www.moodcafe.co.uk—To access free relaxation resources, click Self-Help Material, then Relaxation.

www.getselfhelp.co.uk—On the left-hand side, click Downloads Gallery, then Relaxation, Meditation and Visualisation to get MP3 downloads (there is a small fee to download) and free instruction scripts you can read or print off.

www.stepsforstress.org—Leaflets on coping with stress.

www.eyegaze.tv/health—Self-help relaxation *Stress and Relaxation* DVD for deaf people who use British Sign Language.

www.heartandmindmatters.com—This American website offers a range of services to clients in the United States and provides materials for download that are relevant to cardiac patients.

Index

Note: The italicized *f* and *t* following page numbers refer to figures and tables, respectively.

About the Authors

Morag Thow, PhD, BSc, Dip PE, has been a physiotherapy lecturer specialising in cardiac rehabilitation at Glasgow Caledonian University for over 24 years. She has written two previous titles on cardiac rehabilitation and contributed to another book. She also regularly writes journal articles on cardiac rehabilitation and was a member of the SIGN (Scottish Intercollegiate Guidelines Network) group for Cardiac Rehabilitation 2002. She is a member of BACPR and the Cardiac Rehabilitation Interest Group Scotland.

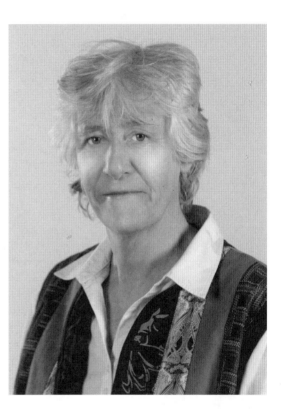

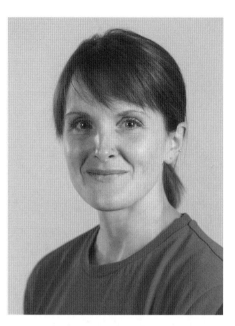

Keri Graham, MSc, BSc, is a chartered physiotherapist who has worked in hospital settings for over 15 years and specialised in cardiac rehabilitation for the past decade. She is a member of the BACPR and Association of Chartered Physiotherapists in Cardiac Rehabilitation (ACPICR) and is a member of the writing group for the ACPICR Standards for Physical Activity and Exercise in the Cardiac Population 2009 and 2012. She is a regular visiting lecturer at Glasgow Caledonian University and is a lead physiotherapist for phase IV cardiac rehabilitation classes in Glasgow.

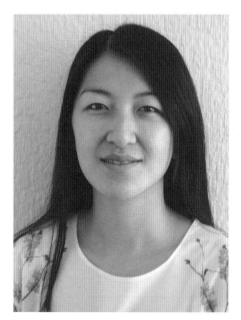

Choi Lee, Bsc, is a qualified dietitian who has specialised in working with cardiac rehabilitation patients since 2008. She is a member of the British Dietetic Association and the Health & Care Professions Council. She is interested in lifestyle interventions in the prevention and treatment of cardiovascular disease and has served as a guest speaker on management and treatment of coronary heart disease as part of the Glasgow University master class series.

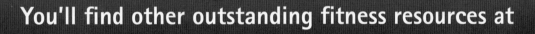
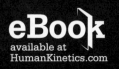